Psychosocial Aspects
of Narcolepsy

Psychosocial Aspects of Narcolepsy

Meeta Goswami, Charles P. Pollak, Felissa L. Cohen,
Michael J. Thorpy, and Neil B. Kavey
Editors

Austin H. Kutscher, *Loss, Grief & Care* Series
Editor-in-Chief

Jill C. Crabtree
Editor for the Foundation of Thanatology

The Haworth Press, Inc.
New York • London

Psychosocial Aspects of Narcolepsy has also been published as *Loss, Grief & Care*, Volume 5, Numbers 3/4 1992.

The Haworth Press, Inc., 10 Alice Street, Binghamton, NY 13904-1580 USA

Library of Congress Cataloging-in-Publication Data

Psychosocial aspects of narcolepsy / Meeta Goswami . . . [et al.], editors; Jill C. Crabtree, editor
  for the Foundation of Thanatology.
      p.   cm.
  "Has also been published as Loss, grief & care, v. 5, nos. 3/4, 1992"–T.p. verso.
  Includes bibliographical references.
  ISBN 0-7890-6047-7 (alk. paper)
  1. Narcolepsy–Psychological aspects. 2. Narcolepsy–Social aspects. I. Goswami, Meeta.
  [DNLM: 1. Narcolepsy–psychology. W1 L0853F v.5 nos. 3/4]
RC549.P78 1992
616.8'498–dc20
DNLM/DLC
for Library of Congress   92-1525
                                                                             CIP

This book is dedicated to the living memory
of Florence and Albert Abelson

Psychosocial Aspects
of Narcolepsy

CONTENTS

Psychosocial Aspects
of Narcolepsy

ABOUT THE EDITORS

Meeta Goswami, PhD, MPH, is Director of the Narcolepsy Institute at the Montefiore Medical Center. She has taught at Columbia University and presented results of her research studies in narcolepsy both nationally and internationally.

Charles P. Pollak, MD, is Head of the Sleep-Wake Disorders Center; Director of the Institute of Chronobiology; and Associate Professor of Neurology and Psychiatry at New York Hospital, Cornell Medical Center.

Felissa L. Cohen, RN, PhD, FAAN, is Director of the Center for Narcolepsy Research, and Professor and Head of the Department of Medical and Surgical Nursing at the College of Nursing of the University of Illinois at Chicago. She is author and co-editor of two books which won *Journal of Nursing* Book of the Year Awards.

Michael J. Thorpy, MD, is Director of the Sleep-Wake Disorders Center at the Montefiore Medical Center and Associate Professor of Neurology at the Albert Einstein College of Medicine. He is editor of *The Handbook of Sleep Disorders* and author of *The Encyclopedia of Sleep and Sleep Disorders.*

Neil B. Kavey, MD, is Associate Clinical Professor of Psychiatry at the College of Physicians and Surgeons, Columbia University, and Associate Attending Psychiatrist at Columbia Presbyterian Medical Center.

Austin H. Kutscher, PhD, is President of The Foundation of Thanatology and Professor of Dentistry (in Psychiatry) at the College of Physicians and Surgeons, Columbia University, New York, New York.

Psychosocial Aspects of Narcolepsy

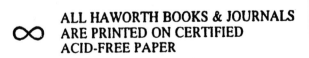

Preface

Although most of us spend approximately one-third of our lives in the sweet repose of sleep, it is only in the past two decades that this valuable and intriguing aspect of human behavior has been the focus of concerted biomedical and psychosocial research.

That sleep has a valuable function is implied in the poem by Eugene Henry Pullen: "Now I lay me down to sleep / I pray the Lord my soul to keep." Sleep is intriguing in that its various benefits still remain relatively unexplored. The recuperative function of sleep has been observed by several writers. The causes and functions of dreams, a subject of much inquiry, remain a mystery.

The intricacies of disruptions in the sleep pattern in various population groups is only beginning to gain the interest of investigators. In this area of research, we have accumulated a somewhat broader base of knowledge about initiating and maintaining sleep, whereas disorders of excessive somnolence are only now emerging as problems worthy of scientific inquiry.

In this context, biomedical aspects of narcolepsy have recently gained the attention of investigators, but little is known about the psychosocial dimensions of this chronic illness. While medications may relieve the physical symptoms of this disorder, the perceived needs and consequences of symptoms on the affected person's feelings, interpersonal relationships, productivity and overall quality of life are relatively unexplored areas.

This volume provides a forum for a wide array of interested professionals to present research findings, clinical studies and theoretical reflections on the psychosocial dimensions of narcolepsy. As such, it is the first text on the psychosocial basis of care of narcolepsy patients. Although the focus is on the human aspects of care, medical aspects have not been neglected. This volume will serve as a valuable resource for all professionals who wish to gain an understanding of narcolepsy and other disorders of excessive daytime sleepiness.

Meeta Goswami, MPH, PhD

Acknowledgment

THE EDITORS WISH to acknowledge the support and encouragement of the Foundation of Thanatology in the preparation of this volume. All royalties from the sale of this book are assigned to the Foundation of Thanatology, a tax exempt, not for profit, public scientific and educational foundation.

Thanatology, a new subspecialty of medicine, is involved in scientific and humanistic inquiries and the application of the knowledge derived therefrom to the subjects of the psychological aspects of dying; reactions to loss, death, and grief; and recovery from bereavement.

The Foundation of Thanatology is dedicated to advancing the cause of enlightened health care for the terminally ill patient and his family. The Foundation's orientation is a positive one based on the philosophy of fostering a more mature acceptance and understanding of death and the problems of grief and the more effective and humane management and treatment of the dying patient and his bereaved family members.

* * *

The publication of this book was supported in part by a grant from the Lucius N. Littauer Foundation.

* * *

Narcolepsy Network is proud as both advocates and activists to have been a co-sponsor of this publication.

SECTION I:
QUALITY OF LIFE ISSUES IN NARCOLEPSY

Life Effects of Narcolepsy:
Measures of Negative Impact,
Social Support,
and Psychological Well-Being

Susan Lines Alaia

Narcolepsy is a chronic neurological disease with multiple symptoms, the primary and most disabling being excessive daytime sleepiness (EDS) (Dement 1976). It has been estimated that narcolepsy affects between two and three people per 1,000 (Regestein 1986). This is more frequent than multiple sclerosis (Broughton and Mamelak 1979). It appears that males have a slightly higher incidence of the disease than females (Billiard 1985). Age of onset is generally between 15 and 30, but it has been found in children as young as five and can begin in the fourth and fifth decades (Passouant and Billiard 1976).

The typical narcoleptic sees numerous physicians over 15 years

Susan Lines Alaia, MSW, resides in Fountain Valley, CA.

before being correctly diagnosed (Scharf et al. 1985). The disease may not be diagnosed "until the patient is elderly as a result of lack of clinical awareness and fluctuations of symptoms" (Quan, Bamford and Beutler 1984, p. 45). There is no cure for this disease, which is generally lifelong following its onset; and only marginal symptomatic relief is available through drug treatment (Broughton and Mamelak 1979).

Broughton and Ghanem (1976) were the first to study systematically the impact of this disease on the life of the patient. They found that individuals with narcolepsy have long personal histories of marked detrimental effects involving interpersonal relationships, employment, education, recreation, and other parameters of everyday life. Subsequent research revealed these effects to be basically the same across cultures (Broughton et al. 1983). Another study showed high levels of psychopathology among narcoleptics, which the investigators considered to be a reaction to the disorder and its effects (Kales et al. 1982). The psychosocial effects of the disease are nonetheless often neglected, and there is a paucity of literature on these aspects of narcolepsy (Regestein 1986).

While there has been some evidence that narcoleptics have little interest in psychotherapy (Broughton and Ghanem 1976), those who have entered into therapy have been interested in resolving the problems they face due to the limitations of the disease as well as dealing with their feelings about being "overly sleepy people" (Regestein 1986, p. 136). Group therapy has also been suggested to help narcoleptics and their families to accept and cope with the disease (Regestein 1986) and has proven to be beneficial (Zarcone and Fuchs 1976).

Cognitive models of stress and coping (Folkman, Schaefer, and Lazarus 1979) emphasize the appraisal of stressful situations and resources available for coping. Observations in a variety of settings have shown that social support contributes to positive adjustment and provides a buffer against the effects of stress (Sarason et al. 1983). Social support is defined by Cobb (1976) as "information leading the subject to believe that he is cared for and loved, esteemed, and a member of a network of mutual obligations" (p. 300).

Schulz and Decker (1985) found a relationship between high levels of social support and high levels of well-being among persons with spinal cord injuries, a chronic condition. The effects of social support on narcolepsy, a chronic condition with pervasive life effects, appears to be a fruitful area of investigation, particularly with respect to depression. There is a high incidence of depression among narcoleptics (Regestein, Reich, and Mufson 1983). Depression and distress have been found to be negatively associated with perceived social support (Barrera 1986).

Despite the psychosocial effects of narcolepsy, a review of the literature reveals a primary focus on etiology, pathophysiological mechanisms, and medications. The purpose of the research described in this paper was to assess the life effects of narcolepsy and the extent to which nondrug treatment methods (such as behavioral/environmental strategies and psychotherapy/support groups) are prescribed. Due to the somewhat conflicting views concerning the interest of narcoleptics in psychotherapy and groups, a needs assessment of this area and related concerns was included. Another area of interest was the relationship between the severity of the negative life effects of the disease and life satisfaction, with a view to determining whether perceived social support mitigates these effects. Specific hypotheses were as follows: (a) negative impact of narcolepsy scores would be inversely correlated with psychological well-being scores; that is, those more highly impacted by narcolepsy would have less psychological well-being; (b) psychological well-being scores would be correlated with social support scores; and (c) social support scores would be inversely correlated with negative impact of narcolepsy.

METHOD

The research involved a national survey of approximately 500 randomly selected members of the American Narcolepsy Association. Data were descriptive, and correlational analyses were conducted to test the relationships among the negative impact of narcolepsy and psychological well-being scores, between social support and psychological well-being, and among social support and negative impact of narcolepsy scores.

Measures

The survey form consisted of 116 items and included a modified version of the Broughton et al. (1981) questionnaire. The negative impact of narcolepsy was defined operationally in terms of number and severity of symptoms; efficacy of medications; and psychosocial impact on employment, education, marital and social relationships, and leisure activities. A modified version of Goodman's (1988) Perceived Social Support Scale operationally defined social support operationally. The Affect-Balance Scale (Bradburn 1969) defined psychological well-being operationally.

Subjects

Narcoleptics were defined operationally as members of the American Narcolepsy Association who indicated that they had both excessive daytime sleepiness or sleep attacks and cataplexy symptoms. Cataplexy is pathognomic of narcolepsy and was therefore required as an auxiliary symptom to ensure that only true narcoleptics were included in the sample. This requirement is in accord with Broughton and Ghanem (1976) who considered this auxiliary symptom to be essential in their narcoleptic sample for sample homogeneity. Survey forms were mailed nationally to 500 ANA members picked at random from the organization's 60,000 members. A total of 146 narcoleptics responded. Of these 146 respondents, 102 had the required combination of symptoms. There were 42 males and 60 females in the sample.

RESULTS

Description of Sample

The 102 subjects ranged in age from 28 to 80, with a mean age of 53.5 and a standard deviation of 11.00. Eight subjects were single, 54 were in their first marriage, 20 were remarried, three were separated, seven were widowed, and two were living with a significant other. The racial composition consisted of 91 subjects who listed themselves as Caucasian, seven as Native American, two as Black, and one as Asian. There were no Hispanics, and one subject did not respond to this question. It was clear from other data that a number of subjects listing themselves as Native American had misunderstood the term. It is probable that all these individuals were Caucasian.

Symptoms

The age at onset of symptoms ranged from 5 to 49. The mean age when symptoms began was 20.6, with a standard deviation of 9.56. Age at diagnosis ranged from 10 to 60, with a mean of 35.8 and a standard deviation of 11.09. Excessive daytime sleepiness (EDS) was the symptom of longest duration, with sleep attacks and cataplexy following by an average of six and four years respectively. The current severity of symptoms was rated using a 4-point scale ranging from 1 (mild) to 4 (most severe). Excessive daytime sleepiness has the highest severity rating mean of 2.5, with a standard deviation of 0.98.

Medication Effectiveness

In this sample, 80 (78.2%) were currently taking medications for some or all of their symptoms. Nineteen were taking medication for EDS; 18 for EDS and cataplexy, 12 for EDS and sleep attacks, 4 for cataplexy, 1 for restless nighttime sleep, and 14 for all of their symptoms. A total of 48% of 100 subjects reported tolerating some symptoms for which medication was available due to undesirable side effects of these drugs. In terms of symptom relief provided by medications, 29.7% of the subjects reported EDS as the symptom most relieved; this symptom was among the top two that were relieved least (26.6%). Cataplexy was slightly higher in the least relieved category at 29.7%.

The degree to which medication improves functioning was rated in three areas: general functioning, driving, and work. Only 2% rated general functioning as greatly improved by medications, but driving and work were rated as greatly improved by 38.6% and 30.0%, respectively. A subscale of these three variables was constructed with a possible range of 0 to 12. The mean score was 7.0 with a standard deviation of 3.45.

Life Effects: Education

Narcolepsy symptoms began before formal education was completed in 61.8% of the respondents. Among these 63 subjects, symptoms were thought to have contributed to poor marks in 64.6%, to embarrassment in 81.8%, to problems with teachers in 48.4%, with parents in 38.1%, and with friends in 37.8%.

Education level attained was scored with a range from 1 (less than twelfth grade) to 6 (post-graduate degree). The mean education level was 3.0 with a standard deviation of 1.35. This score indicates that the average education level included some college/university credits but no degree.

Life Effects: Driving

There were 95 drivers among this sample. Sleepiness was reported a problem when driving by 78% of the sample. Before diagnosis and treatment, 29% reported having had accidents due to their symptoms, and 74.2% reported having had near accidents. A subscale of driving problems was constructed with a range of 3 (least problems) to 6 (most problems). The mean score was 4.9 with a standard deviation of 2.07.

Life Effects: Work/Career

In terms of the effects of the disease on the work/career chosen and the difficulties encountered, nearly 85% of respondents felt that their symptoms had reduced their job performance and 15% had become permanently disabled by their disease.

Current employment was reported by 64.4%. Subjects reported that excessive daytime sleepiness is the most problematic symptom.

Feelings of competency in their jobs were rated on a 4-point scale from 1 (not at all) to 4 (great). The mean score was 2.7 with a standard deviation of 1.46. Their overall level of satisfaction with current job or career was rated on a 5-point scale from 1 (not satisfied) to 5 (very satisfied). The mean score was 2.9 with a standard deviation of 1.89.

Life Effects: Leisure Activities

Regular exercise was reported by 36.6% of the respondents, and 77.4% indicated that they were physically fit. A majority (70.6%) reported that their symptoms interfered with their enjoyment of recreational activities. Symptoms had caused 62.8% to give up their favorite leisure activities. A subscale of these variables was constructed with a possible range of 4 (least problems) to 8 (most problems). The mean score was 6.1 with a standard deviation of 1.13.

Life Effects: Interpersonal Relationships

There were four questions concerning interpersonal relationships. One question was of a general nature and three were specific to intimate relationships. A subscale of these variables was constructed with a range of 1 to 5. Total composite score range was 4 to 20. The highest mean score of 3.9 was obtained for the rating of their current marital or intimate relationship being supportive and sympathetic.

Life Effects: Sexual Life

Of the 95 subjects who responded to the question, 36.1% reported that narcolepsy had been associated with a decrease in their sexual drive. The frequency distribution for responses regarding particular aspects of sexual functioning was calculated. Impotence in males was the most widely reported problem. While 15.8% rated the effects of their symptoms on the quality of their sexual life as severely negative, 45.3% reported no negative effect.

A rating of overall sexual satisfaction was obtained with a 5-point scale ranging from 1 (not satisfied) to 5 (very satisfied). The mean score was 3.1 with a standard deviation of 1.58.

Social Support

Data From Goodman's (1988) Perceived Social Support Subscale was examined. Scores ranged from 1 (Definitely no) to 5 (Definitely yes). The highest mean value obtained was 2.9, for knowing someone who understands their difficulties. A composite social support score was calculated, with a possible range of 9 to 45; the mean was 20.7 with a standard deviation of 8.50.

Psychological Well-Being

Scores for the five positive affect scale questions and the five negative affect questions from Bradburn's (1969) Affect Balance Scale were summed separately. The difference between the two scores was computed as the indicator of each subject's psychological well-being. A constant of 20 was added to each of the well-being scores to eliminate negative values. The mean and standard deviation for each of these three subscales were computed. These data are presented in Table 1. The first two subscales had a possible range of 5 to 25. The summary subscale had a possible range of 0 to 40.

HYPOTHESIZED RELATIONSHIPS

An 11 × 11 correlation matrix was constructed to examine the relationships among the measures of negative impact of narcolepsy, social support, and psychological well-being. The matrix consisted of: the symptom severity subscale, the driving problems subscale, the job satisfaction rating, the leisure limitations subscale, the interpersonal relations subscale, the medication effectiveness subscale, the social support subscale, and Bradburn's (1969) positive affect, negative affect, and affect balance summary subscales.

TABLE 1. Mean Responses to Bradburn's (1969) Affect Balance Scale

Subscale	M	SD
Positive Affect	17.9	5.90
Negative Affect	15.0	5.34
Affect Balance Summary Score	22.5	9.18

Note. N = 100. The first two scales had a range of 5 to 25; the last had a range of 0 to 40. A constant of 20 was added to the Affect Balance Summary Scores to eliminate negative values.

Pearson correlation coefficients were computed to test the hypothesized relationships. The correlation matrix is displayed in Table 2. Hypothesis 1 predicted that negative impact of narcolepsy scores would be inversely correlated with psychological well-being, defined by Bradburn's (1969) subscales. This hypothesis was supported in some areas of life but not in others. As expected, there were correlations among the affect balance summary score and interpersonal relations ($r = .25, p < .05$), sex satisfaction ($r = .46$, $p < .001$), job satisfaction ($r = .34, p < .01$), and leisure limitations ($r = -.32, p < .01$). Expected correlations were found between the positive affect score and sex satisfaction ($r = .41, p < .001$) and job satisfaction ($r = .34, p < .001$). Expected correlations were found between the negative affect score and interpersonal relations ($r = -.39, p < .001$), sex satisfaction ($r = -.33$, $p < .01$), job satisfaction ($r = -.22, p < .05$), and leisure limitations ($r = .34, p < .01$). The expected correlation among the affect balance subscales and the symptom severity subscale was not found. There was also no expected correlation between symptom severity and sex or job satisfaction. Correlations were found, as expected, between symptom severity and leisure limitations ($r = .36, p < .001$) and driving problems ($r = .26, p < .05$). Other correlations included driving problems and leisure limitations ($r = .24, p < .05$), interpersonal relationships and sex satisfaction ($r = .26, p < .05$), and job satisfaction and sex satisfaction ($r = .39$, $p < .001$).

Hypotheses 2 and 3 involved Goodman's (1988) Perceived Social Support subscale. It was predicted that social support would be correlated with psychological well-being, defined by Bradburn's (1969) subscales. It was also predicted that social support scores would be inversely correlated with negative impact of narcolepsy scores. Neither correlation was found.

The overall support rating is an item from Goodman's (1988) subscale. A correlation matrix was constructed to analyze the relationship among the overall support rating, the marital satisfaction rating from the interpersonal relationship subscale, and the five positive affect items. A similar correlation matrix was constructed to analyze the relationships among ratings of overall support, marital satisfaction, and the five negative affect items. Pearson correlation

Table 2. Correlations Involving Affect Balance Subscales, Social Support, and Indices of Narcolepsy Life Effects

	Positive Affect	Negative Affect	Affect Balance	Social Support	Inter-personal	Sex Satis-faction	Job Satis-faction	Symptom Severity	Leisure Limits	Driving Problems	Meds Effec-tiveness
Positive Affect	1.00	–	–	–	–	–	–	–	–	–	–
Negative Affect	-.20	1.00	–	–	–	–	–	–	–	–	–
Affect Balance	.83***	.62***	1.00	–	–	–	–	–	–	–	–
Social Support	.16	-.07	.16	1.00	–	–	–	–	–	–	–
Inter-personal	.07	-.39***	.25*	.21	1.00	–	–	–	–	–	–
Sex Satis-faction	.41***	-.33**	.46***	.11	.26*	1.00	–	–	–	–	–
Job Satis-faction	.34**	-.22*	.34**	-.06	-.01	.39***	1.00	–	–	–	–
Symptom Severity	.06	.08	.03	-.01	-.20	-.13	-.13	1.00	–	–	–
Leisure Limits	-.16	.34**	-.32**	-.08	-.15	-.17	-.08	.36***	1.00	–	–
Driving Problems	.05	.17	.01	-.01	-.19	-.06	-.08	.26*	.24*	1.00	–
Meds Effec-tiveness	.14	-.20	.16	-.04	.07	.09	.37***	-.04	.02	-.04	1.00

*p < .05, **p < .01, ***p < .001

coefficients were computed. The overall support rating was highly correlated with the marital satisfaction rating ($r = .30, p < .01$) and with two items from the positive affect scale, recently complimented ($r = .30, p < .01$) and pleased about accomplishment ($r = .26, p < .01$). The overall support rating was correlated with 2 items from the negative affect subscale, with feeling depressed ($r = .24, p < .05$) and feeling lonely ($r = .27, p < .01$).

Coping Assistance

The needs assessment section of the questionnaire was tabulated. As expected, most narcoleptics had not received coping assistance from their physicians beyond medication prescriptions. There was a clear interest in both professional mental health assistance and support groups. A majority (67.3%) would currently see a therapist who was well-informed about narcolepsy, and 83.6% would join a support group.

In terms of issues these subjects would bring to a mental health professional meeting the above criterion, coping strategies were selected by 72.3%. Nearly half (47.5) selected personal feelings about having narcolepsy and its impact on their lives.

DISCUSSION

In view of the difficulties in intimate relationships reported (Broughton and Ghanem 1976; Broughton 1981), this sample seems to have a high number of individuals who were still in their first marriage. With the exception of the seven who were widowed, only 11 appeared not to be living in an intimate relationship.

The age of onset of symptoms was as described by Passouant and Billiard (1976). These subjects had lived with their disease an average of 33 years. Nearly one half of this period was without the benefit of a diagnosis; and this is a typical pattern among narcoleptics (Scharf et al. 1985).

Excessive daytime sleepiness was the longest term symptom. It also had the highest severity rating. The refractory nature of this symptom is evident in its high severity rating despite the fact that most subjects were on medication, that it was rated as the most relieved by medication, and that these ratings of severity were taking the effect of the drugs into account. It was also second only to cataplexy in the "least relieved" category. The present study is in accord with the literature concerning the variability among narcoleptics in terms of symptom onset and severity (Baker et al. 1986) and the efficacy of drug treatment (Broughton and Mamelak 1979).

A majority obtained some relief from symptoms with medication, and there was a positive relationship between medication effectiveness and job satisfaction. There was also, however, a large number of individuals who obtain minimal or no improvement with drug therapy. Nearly half reported tolerating some symptoms because drug side-effects were less tolerable than the symptoms. Some specific side-effects mentioned included feeling nervous, severe headaches, blood pressure problems, and heart damage. Heart problems were mentioned by several subjects. One described her's as "enlarged and damaged and too fast" due to narcolepsy medications. Another described his heart problems due to narcolepsy medications and the death of his father, also narcoleptic, whose fatal heart attack he attributed to stimulant medication.

On the other hand, there were subjects who added very favorable comments about the effectiveness of drug treatment. One woman described all of her symptoms as improved and added, "Gamma [gamma-hydroxybutyrate], in particular, is a 'miracle' drug for narcoleptics."

Getting medication was reported as a problem by several. These difficulties were similar to those reported by others (Broughton and Ghanem 1976; Rogers 1984). They involved pharmacists who refused to fill prescriptions, some using derisive language concerning the patients being drug addicts and "speed freaks." Others had had problems with physicians who were ignorant about the disease and refused to prescribe the required medication. One respondent had a psychiatrist who insisted the disease was psychogenic and continued to do so, and refused to prescribe medication on that basis, even after being presented with recent research to the contrary.

Many of the negative life effects reported by others, particularly by Broughton and his associates (Broughton, and Ghanem 1976; Broughton et al. 1981; Broughton, Guberman and Roberts 1984), were found in the present study. Among those whose symptoms began before their formal education was completed, the same negative reports were given concerning poor marks, social embarrassment, and interpersonal problems. There were many poignant comments from subjects concerning living with narcolepsy. One woman wrote that memories of her school years were "sad" and full of comments from teachers that she was not "working up to my potential." She went on to say that, "Concentration was a narcotic. My mind fell in and out of consciousness as I studied." In retrospect, she said she realizes her average grades in college were an accomplishment, but at the time she was "so caught up in my struggle to emulate my older sister, I only remembered that I had lost the struggle."

The reported difficulties in driving a car were similar in most respects to those found previously (Broughton and Ghanem 1976; Broughton et al. 1981), but there were differences as well. Among the questions on the original survey (Broughton and Ghanem 1976, p. 205) were the following concerning accidents when driving: (a) "Has Narcolepsy led to an accident?" and (b) "Has Narcolepsy led to frequent near accidents?" Other questions asked for their severity rating of accidents and the kinds of symptoms experienced while driving. These investigators found their results so "discouraging" that they concluded that "driving licenses should probably be suspended for most, if not all, narcoleptics" (Broughton and Ghanem 1976, pp. 205-206).

These questions appeared to be open to some interpretation by respondents. Affirmative responses could refer to subjects' current difficulties or they could refer to circumstances before diagnosis and treatment, e.g., has Narcolepsy (ever) led to these situations. To attempt to assess both the past and present situation, the questions were changed to clearly indicate difficulties prior to diagnosis and treatment as well as the degree to which medications solved driving problems. Results suggest that narcoleptics driving problems are resolved to a considerable degree when they can tolerate medications. Unsolicited comments from both medicated and unmedicated subjects indicated high levels of awareness and concern about safety while driving. Some indicated that they only drove short distances, others only drove in the morning when they were alert, and many had diverse strategies for coping with driving. These included ice-packs on the back of their necks, cold drinks, no eating before driving (especially no "sweets"), stopping at intervals to get exercise, keeping the car interior cool, and singing along with the radio. It seems reasonable to conclude that narcoleptics are aware of any difficulties they have, have developed coping strategies, and in general pose no greater risk behind the wheel than anyone else.

One of the difficulties reported concerning driving was the confusion between epilepsy and narcolepsy on the part of Departments of Motor Vehicles in some states. One subject attached to her survey a copy (with her name removed) of a letter she had written to the agency in her state attempting to educate them. An excerpt from it seems to sum up her frustration and that of others in getting a medical release to drive:

> One of your forms . . . lists narcolepsy as one of the "kinds" of "epilepsy!" With such blatant lack of knowledge, is it any wonder that one of my doctors told me I should not have mentioned my narcolepsy to you?

A positive relationship was found between driving problems and severity of symptoms. There was no relationship found between driving problems and the medication effectiveness subscale. This seems to indicate that medication alone is not enough to cope and may be behind some of the other coping strategies employed.

There was a strong positive relationship between driving problems and leisure activity limitations. This represents quite a negative life effect in our car-oriented society.

Leisure activity limitations were also strongly related to symptom severity and the negative affect subscale. Narcoleptics' ability to engage in their favorite activities is clearly affected by their disease.

Narcolepsy has had a definite impact on the ability to fulfill the important role responsibilities relating to jobs or careers. Excessive daytime sleepiness, cataplexy, memory, and concentration problems were identified as resulting in reduced job performance, accidents, worry about job loss, and both temporary and permanent disability. These findings are in accord with previous studies

(Broughton and Ghanem 1976; Broughton et al. 1981; Broughton, Guberman and Roberts 1984).

The results from questions developed for the present study showed that many individuals had had to change their career plans and actual employment due to their symptoms. Some of the jobs given up were engineer, teacher, flight engineer, journalist, salesperson, accountant, railroad engineer, truck driver, and secretary. One subject reported selling his business because he could no longer "cope with employees." Other personal comments included being stuck in a job because advancement required more education, which the subject could not handle due to sleepiness; being afraid to admit to the disease because of stigma and fear of job loss and actual termination of employment because of it.

Job satisfaction ratings averaged at about the mid point and job competency ratings were slightly above. The variability among the subjects was high, indicating that there were many on each of the extreme ends of the scale. Those at the higher, more positive end are in accord with McMahon and others (1982). They found that compared to other disabled individuals, narcoleptics had above average scores in vocational self-actualization, economic security, and economic self-esteem. Several who reported the highest levels of job satisfaction indicated that they had found jobs in which they were physically active, could take short naps, or arrange their schedules to coincide with their more alert periods of the day. Several were self-employed. The flexibility required in a job to utilize some of these coping strategies may be an important missing factor among those whose job satisfaction was lower.

The most significant factor in job satisfaction, however, appears to be the efficacy of drug therapy. There was a strong positive relationship between job satisfaction and medication effectiveness. The work/career area was the only life-effects area which demonstrated a relationship with the effectiveness of medications.

The importance of job satisfaction to psychological well-being is demonstrated by (a) the positive relationship between positive affect and job satisfaction and (b) the inverse relationship between negative affect and job satisfaction. These findings seem to support the view that psychological well-being is linked to an individual's ability to meet important role obligations (Thoits 1985).

Interpersonal relationships appear to have been negatively affected by narcolepsy. Replies to the question concerning whether or not their symptoms had been a source of difficulty in their marriage or intimate relationship were somewhat equivocal, averaging between "Probably yes" and "Not sure." Their replies to whether or not their symptoms were a prime factor in the break up of such relationships was more clearly affirmative, averaging between "Definitely yes" and "Probably yes." The most positive rating was given to the question concerning current intimate relationships being supportive, just short of a "Probably yes" reply. The difference in the average response between difficulties in the marriage and the supportive nature of current relationships may indicate that at least some of these individuals have learned how to resolve or cope with these difficulties.

There was a strong inverse relationship between the negative affect subscale and the interpersonal relationship scale. This seems to suggest that those individuals with a high degree of negative affect are not in supportive relationships or those who are in supportive intimate relationships do not have a high degree of negative affect.

A positive relationship was not found between positive affect and intimate relationships. This may indicate that those with a high degree of positive affect are that way whether they are in supportive relationships or not; their affect is related to other factors. That supportive interpersonal relations are correlated with negative affect but not positive suggests that such social support can help prevent negative feelings but may not result in positive feelings. This reflects the literature that emphasizes that close relationships may buffer stress but may also contribute to stress (Coyne and DeLongis 1986).

There was a positive relationship between the interpersonal relationship subscale and the sexual satisfaction scale. This suggests that those who are in supportive intimate relationships have high levels of sexual satisfaction. Sexual satisfaction was strongly positively related to positive affect and strongly inversely related to negative affect. The importance of sexual satisfaction to psychological well-being is suggested. The strong positive relationship between job and sexual satisfaction was not predicted. This may suggest that common factors contribute to both types of satisfaction.

The social support averages on each item of the Goodman (1988) scale were quite low. None of the scores reached above the mid point. These scores seem to represent the sentiments voiced in many ways by the narcoleptics in this study. The comments of one are representative:

> Having narcolepsy has been a lonely experience. Only recently have I come to know others with it. A support group through the 40 + years would have helped me cope so much. Family and friends have been understanding, but they don't really 'know' my feelings and frustration . . . only persons with it [narcolepsy] can understand.

These individuals feel their situation is beyond the ability of their support system to comprehend. The failure to find a relationship between social support and any of the life-effect or affect measures suggests that social support, as a coping strategy for those aspects of their lives related to narcolepsy, is not available. It could be, however, that the negative life effects of narcolepsy are such that perceptions of social support are distorted. This would support Barrera's (1986) view that perceptions of social support decrease as life stresses increase. He also found that depression had a negative effect on perceived social support, and this was demonstrated by Procidano and Heller (1983). The depression evident in this sample may be adversely effecting their social support perceptions.

An item from the social support subscale asks for an agreement rating with the statement, "Overall, I feel satisfied with the support I have received from others as I cope with Narcolepsy." The positive relationship found between this item and the overall rating of current intimate relationships suggests the importance of the marital relationship as social support (Lieberman 1986; Monroe et al. 1986). The relationship between this overall support rating and feelings of depression and loneliness suggests the impact of this void in the lives of narcoleptics.

The literature is replete with findings of depression in narcoleptics (Broughton et al. 1981; Broughton and Ghanem 1976; Krishnan et al. 1984; Regestein, Reich and Mufson 1983; Reynolds et al. 1982). The present study has found such depression, and it has suggested areas of living related to it and independent from it. Depression, as defined by the negative affect subscale (Bradburn 1969), was related to interpersonal problems, sexual and job satisfaction, and limitations on leisure activities. These represent the major areas of everyday living. It was not, however, related to symptom severity. This seems likely to be due to the pervasiveness of the disease; that is, the symptoms at any level are deleterious. Depression was not related to medication effectiveness either, although the inverse correlation approached significance. This seems to be representative of the effects of medication. While helpful, they "certainly do not normalize" the quality of life for narcoleptics (Broughton et al. 1983, p. 103).

An important function of support groups is their ability to normalize the feelings and experiences of group members. The failure of physicians to recommend support groups, or other kinds of psychosocial assistance, is an area of particular concern. Contrary to studies showing a lack of interest among narcoleptics in psychotherapy (Broughton and Ghanem 1976; Dement et al. 1976), a large majority of the narcoleptics in the present study were interested in therapy and support groups.

While support groups generally attract women members (Taylor et al. 1986), there was no apparent difference between the males' and females' interest in support groups in the sample. Based on their comments, self-help groups for this population should be prepared to integrate two types of self-help groups (Levy 1979), those in which members share a common stress-producing life-circumstance and those in which members are concerned with enhancing self-esteem and improving their situation through educational and political activities. The former type provide the environment "akin to therapy" (Lieberman 1986, p. 464), and the latter provide a vehicle for advocacy. The dearth of such groups for this sample was a clear problem, as evidenced by their many personal comments to that effect and expressed interest in them.

One of the possible limitations of this study is the self-selected sample of narcoleptics who belong to the ANA. Perhaps such individuals are different in some important way than those who are not members. It could be argued that ANA members in general are more well-informed about their disease and therefore aware of the Association. This may indicate a generally higher degree of resources (socioeconomic, intellectual, or emotional). On the other hand, their membership may be argued as evidence of a more problematic adjustment and a greater need for resources. There is no information in this study to support either viewpoint. The same kinds of arguments could be made concerning the self-selection of those who actually responded to the survey. As the results are consistent with the literature, this sample appears to be representative in general. A possible limitation is the few minority members in the sample. Broughton et al. (1983) found the effects of the disease to be consistent across cultural/racial boundaries. While there is no reason to suspect the disease affects different racial or ethnic groups differently, Broughton et al. (1983) were studying members of the majority cultures in these countries. The deleterious effects of the disease among members of racial or ethnic minorities could be even greater. These individuals are already stigmatized and disadvantaged because of their minority status. If members of the majority culture report being accused of being lazy, of having difficulty getting stimulant medication, and suffering the other socioeconomic and emotional effects of the disease, one can only imagine how much worse it could be for minority racial and ethnic groups. Narcolepsy among these groups may be a fruitful area for future investigation.

Some older narcoleptics have been reported as experiencing a worsening of symptoms with age (Montplaisir and Godbout 1986). The literature suggests that sleep disorders are exacerbated among the elderly by other medical problems (Dement, Miles and Carskadon 1982). Nineteen of the 102 subjects in this sample were elderly (at least 65 years old). While there were no questions specific to the effect of aging on symptoms, a few of these elderly subjects commented that their symptoms had lessened over the years. One said that her experience with the disease was "older is better." These unusual findings may simply be due to the idiosyncratic nature of narcolepsy. Passouant and Billiard (1976) have stated that a general evolutionary pattern for the disease has been difficult to determine. The experience of these elderly narcoleptics may, however, be due to other factors which, if known, could be useful in treating the disease among the elderly. This may be an important area for future study.

Another area for investigation is suggested by the apparent lack of relatedness between positive affect and interpersonal relationships and social support. It would be helpful in treating narcoleptics to know if there are individual differences that contribute to a relatively good adjustment to this pervasive disease, whether it is a matter of personality characteristics, cognitive factors, unique coping strategies, self-esteem factors, or perhaps some kinds of social support not identified in this study.

REFERENCES

Baker, T. L., C. Guilleminault, G. Nino-Murcia, and W. C. Dement. 1986. "Comparative Polysomnographic Study of Narcolepsy and Idiopathic Central Nervous System Hypersomnia." *Sleep* 9(1):232-242.

Barrera, M. Jr. 1986. "Distinctions Between Social Support Concepts, Measures, and Models." *American Journal of Community Psychology* 14:413-445.

Billiard, M. 1986. "Narcolepsy: Clinical Features and Aetiology." *Annals Clinical Research* 17(5):220-226.

Bradburn, N. B. 1969. *The Structure of Psychological Well-Being*. Chicago: Aldine.

Broughton, R. and Ghanem, Q. 1976. "The Impact of Compound Narcolepsy on the Life of the Patient." In C. Guilleminault, W. C. Dement, and P. Passouant, eds. *Narcolepsy*. New York: Spectrum, pp. 201-220.

Broughton, R., and M. Mamelak. 1979. "The Treatment of Narcolepsy-Cataplexy with Nocturnal Gamma-Hydroxybutyrate." *Canadian Journal of Neurological Science* 6:1-6.

Broughton, R., Q. Ghanem, Y. Hishikawa, Y. Sugita, S. Nevsimalova, and B. Roth. 1983. "Life Effects of Narcolepsy: Relationship to Geographic Origin (North American, Asian, or European) and to Other Patient and Illness Variables." *Canadian Journal of Neurological Sciences* 10(2):100-104.

Broughton, R. J., A. Guberman, and J. Roberts. 1984. "Comparison of the Psychosocial Effects of Epilepsy and Narcolepsy/Cataplexy: A Controlled Study." *Epilepsia* 25:423433.

Cobb, S. 1976. "Social Support: as a Moderator of Life Stress." *Psychosomatic Medicine* 38:300-314.

Coyne, J., C., and A. DeLongis. 1986. "Going Beyond Social Support: The Role of Social Relationships in Adaptation." *Journal of Consulting and Clinical Psychology* 54:454-460.

Dement, W. C. 1976. "Daytime Sleepiness and Sleep 'Attacks.'" In C. Guilleminault, W. C. Dement, and P. Passouant, eds. *Narcolepsy*. New York: Spectrum, pp. 17-42.

Dement, W. C., M. A. Carskadon, C. Guilleminault, V. P. Zarcone, Jr. 1976. "Narcolepsy: Diagnosis and Treatment." *Primary Care* 3:609-623.

Folkman, S., C. Schaefer, and R. S. Lazarus. 1979. "Cognitive Processes as

Mediators of Stress and Coping." In V. Hamilton and D. M. Warburton, eds. *Human Stress and Cognition*. Chilchester, England: Wiley, pp. 265-298.

Goodman, C. 1988. *Perceived Social Support Scale* (Unpublished scale), California State University, Long Beach, Department of Social Work.

Kales, A., C. R. Soldatos, E. O. Bixler, A. Caldwell, R. J. Cadieux, J. M. Verrechio, and J. D. Kales. 1982. "Narcolepsy-Cataplexy II. Psychosocial Consequences and Associated Psychopathology." *Archives of Neurology* 39(3): 169-171.

Krishnan, R. R., M. R. Volow, P. P. Miller, and S. T. Carwile. 1984. "Narcolepsy: Preliminary Retrospective Study of Psychiatric and Psychosocial Aspects." *American Journal of Psychiatry* 141:428-431.

Levy, L. H. 1979. "Processes and Activities in Groups." In M. A. Lieberman and L. D. Borman, eds. *Self-Help Groups for Coping with Crisis: Origins, Members, Processes, and Impact*. San Francisco: Jossey-Bass, pp. 164-181.

Lieberman, M. A. 1986. "Social Supports – the Consequences of Psychologizing: A Commentary." *Journal of Consulting and Clinical Psychology* 54:461-465.

McMahon, B. T., J. K. Walsh, K. Sexton, and S. A. Smitson. 1982. "Need Satisfaction in Narcolepsy." *Rehabilitation Literature* 43(3-4):82-85.

Monroe, S. M., E. J. Bromet, M. M. Connell, and S. C. Steiner. 1986. "Social Support, Life Events, and Depressive Symptoms: A One-Year Prospective Study." *Journal of Consulting and Clinical Psychology* 54:424-431.

Montplaisir, J. and R. Godbout. 1986. "Nocturnal Sleep of Narcoleptic Patients: Revisited." *Sleep* 9(1):159-161.

Passouant, P. and M. Billiard. 1976. "The Evolution of Narcolepsy with Age." In C. Guilleminault, W. C. Dement, and P. Passouant, eds. *Narcolepsy*. New York: Spectrum, pp. 179-196.

Procidano, M. E. and K. Heller. 1983. "Measures of Perceived Social Support from Friends and from Family: Three Validation Studies." *American Journal of Community Psychology* 11(1):1-25.

Quan, S. F., C. R. Bamford, and L. E. Beutler. 1984. "Sleep Disturbances in the Elderly." *Geriatrics* 39(9):42-47.

Regestein, Q. R. 1986. "Therapy of Narcolepsy." In *Current Psychiatric Therapies*, pp. 129-138.

Regestein, Q. R., P. Reich, and M. J. Mufson. 1983. "Narcolepsy: An Initial Clinical Approach." *Journal of Clinical Psychiatry* 44(5):166-172.

Rogers, A. E. 1984. "Problems and Coping Strategies Identified by Narcoleptic Patients." *Journal of Neurosurgical Nursing* 16:326-334.

Sarason, I. G., H. M. Levine, R. B. Basham, and B. R. Sarason. 1983. "Assessing Social Support: The Social Support Questionnaire." *Journal of Personality and Social Psychology* 44:127-139.

Scharf, M. B., D. Brown, M. Woods, L. Brown, and J. Horowitz. 1985. "The Effects and Effectiveness of Gamma-Hydroxybutyrate in Patients with Narcolepsy." *Journal of Clinical Psychiatry* 46(6):222-225.

Schulz, R., and S. Decker. 1985. "Long-Term Adjustment to Physical Disability:

The Role of Social Support, Perceived Control, and Self-Blame." *Journal of Personality and Social Psychology* 48:1162-1172.

Taylor, S. E., R. L. Falke, S. J. Shoptaw, and R. R. Lichtman. 1986. "Social Support, Support Groups, and the Cancer Patient." *Journal of Consulting and Clinical Psychology* 54:608-615.

Thoits, P. A. 1985. "Social Support and Psychological Well-Being: Theoretical Possibilities." In I. G. Sarason and B. R. Sarason, eds. *Social Support: Theory, Research, and Applications*. Boston: Martin Nijhoff, pp. 51-72.

Zarcone, V. P. Jr., and H. E. Fuchs. 1976. "Psychiatric Disorders and Narcolepsy." In C. Guilleminault, W. C. Dement, and P. Passouant, eds. *Narcolepsy*. New York: Spectrum, pp. 231-256.

The Quality of Life
of Persons with Narcolepsy

Carol E. Ferrans
Felissa L. Cohen
Karen M. Smith

Research on narcolepsy has focused primarily on pathophysiological mechanisms and treatment, rather than on its effects on everyday life. An exception is the group of studies performed by Broughton and his associates (Broughton and Ghanem 1974; Broughton, Ghanem, Hishikawa, Sugita, Nevsimalova, and Roth 1981; Broughton, Ghanem, Hishikawa, Sugita, Nevsimalova, and Roth 1983; Broughton, Guberman, and Roberts 1984), which demonstrated that the symptoms of narcolepsy have a significant detrimental impact on socioeconomic and other aspects of life. This study builds upon and extends these studies. The purpose of this study was to assess the quality of life of persons who have narcolepsy.

Carol E. Ferrans, RN, PhD, is affiliated with the Center for Narcolepsy Research, College of Nursing, University of Illinois at Chicago, Chicago, IL. Felissa L. Cohen, RN, PhD, FAAN, is Director, Center for Narcolepsy Research, and Professor of Medical/Surgical Nursing, College of Nursing, University of Illinois at Chicago, Chicago, IL. Karen M. Smith, PhD, is Senior Research Specialist, Center for Narcolepsy Research, College of Nursing, University of Illinois at Chicago, Chicago, IL.

This research was supported in part by Mr. J. A. Piscopo, founder and retired Chairman of the Board of Directors of Pansophic Systems, Inc. The authors would like to thank the American Narcolepsy Association for its assistance with the data collection for this study.

METHOD

Sample

The sample consisted of 539 persons with narcolepsy. A broad span of ages was represented. Ages ranged from 20 to 97 years, with a mean age of 52.57 years (SD = 12.83). Slightly less than half of the sample were males (43.8%). Regarding race, the sample was almost entirely white (93.8%). Only 3.2% were black, 2.1% were Native American, and 1.0% were Latino, Oriental or other. Sixty-nine percent were married, 16.4% were divorced or separated, 6.9% were widowed, and 7.8% were never married. The sample was well educated. Only 11.4% had not completed high school, 21.0% had completed high school, 36.1% had some college or trade school, and 31.4% had college degrees. The majority were working either full- (41.6%) or part-time (12.1%). Twenty-one percent were retired, 10.6% were housewives, 9.7% were disabled, 3.5% were unemployed, and 1.3% were students. Regarding total family income, 5.1% had incomes of less than $5,000 per year, 8.5% had incomes of $5,000-9,000, 11.0% had $10,000-14,999, 22.8% had $15,000-24,000, 15.7% had $25,000-34,000, and 36.9% had $35,000 or more.

Instruments

Quality of Life Index – Narcolepsy Version. Subjective quality of life was measured by the Narcolepsy Version of the Quality of Life Index (QLI) (Ferrans 1990; Ferrans and Powers 1985). For this instrument, quality of life is conceptualized as "a person's sense of well-being that stems from satisfaction or dissatisfaction with the areas of life that are important to him/her" (Ferrans 1990, p. 15). The instrument consists of 74 items. It has two parts: the first measures how satisfied a person is with many aspects of life, and the second measures how important those same aspects of life are. Subjects respond to items on 6-point Likert scales, ranging from very satisfied to very dissatisfied for Part 1 items and from very important to very unimportant for Part 2 items.

Scores are calculated by weighting the satisfaction items with importance items. This weighting produces scores that reflect how satisfied or dissatisfied the person is with the aspects of life that he or she values. Overall quality of life scores are calculated, as well as four subscale scores. The four subscales reflect quality of life in the areas of health and functioning, the social and economic domain, the psychological/spiritual domain, and family. Overall scores and subscale scores range from 0 to 30, with higher scores indicating better quality of life.

Reliability and validity of the QLI has been established by Ferrans (1990) and Ferrans and Powers (1985). Internal consistency reliability has been supported by coefficient alphas ranging from .90 to .95 for the entire QLI and alphas of .90, .84, .93, and .66 for the health and functioning, social and economic, psychological/ spiritual, and family subscales, respectively. Test-retest reliability has been found to be .87 and .81 with two-week and one-month intervals. Concurrent validity was supported by correlations of .65, .75, and .80 between the QLI and a measure of overall life satisfaction. Support for construct validity was provided by significantly higher mean QLI scores for subjects who had less pain, less depression, and were coping better with stress.

Additional information on quality of life. Questions were developed for the study to obtain additional information regarding the four life domains of health and functioning, social and economic aspects, psychological/spiritual aspects, and family. These questions are described in the "Results" section.

Procedure

Subjects (N = 833) were selected randomly from a mailing list of the American Narcolepsy Association (N = 1666). The list covered 13 states that compose the midsection of the United States, ranging from the northern to southern boundaries of the country. The states were Minnesota, Wisconsin, Michigan, Iowa, Illinois, Indiana, Missouri, Kentucky, Tennessee, Arkansas, Louisiana, Mississippi, and Alabama. Questionnaires were mailed to subjects' homes. The cover letter and questionnaire made clear that respondents must have been diagnosed with narcolepsy to participate. Two follow-up questionnaires were sent to nonrespondents. Of the

783 persons who were eligible and locatable by mail, 539 returned the questionnaire, which represented a 68.8% response rate.

RESULTS

Quality of Life Index

The mean QLI score for overall quality of life was 19.14 (SD = 5.21). This score was compared with that of a healthy group of subjects (M = 21.67, SD = 3.67) from a previous study, which used the general population version of the QLI. The overall, quality of life of the narcolepsy group was significantly lower than that of the healthy group (t (605) = 5.58, p < .005).

To determine which areas contributed most positively or negatively to quality of life, subscale scores for the QLI were calculated. The mean scores were 17.66 (SD = 6.09), 19.39 (SD = 5.22), 19.99 (SD = 6.64), and 22.84 (SD = 6.67), for the health and functioning, social and economic, psychological/spiritual, and family subscales, respectively. A repeated measures ANOVA revealed significant differences among the subscales (F (3,1524) = 173.38, p < .0001). A Tukey test was used to identify the source of the differences (critical difference = .716, p < .01). It was found that *all* means were significantly different from each other, except for social/economic and psychological/spiritual. Thus, quality of life was found to be highest in the family domain, followed by the psychological/spiritual domain, and social and economic domain. Quality of life was lowest in the area of health and functioning.

Similar results were found when subjects were asked how satisfied they were with their lives in general. This was rated on a scale from 1 (very dissatisfied) to 6 (very satisfied). The mean response was 4.36 (SD = 1.48), which indicated that subjects were only slightly satisfied with their lives.

Health and Functioning

Table 1 reports the percentages of subjects who were troubled either moderately or a great deal by the symptoms typically associated with narcolepsy. The majority reported difficulty with daytime drowsiness, sleep attacks, and restless nighttime sleep. Subjects also were asked which activities brought on symptoms of narcolepsy or made them worse. As can be seen in Table 2, the most frequently reported activities were monotonous activities, reading, too little sleep, boredom, excitement, and stress.

Subjects were asked whether their memory had remained the same, improved, or worsened since developing narcolepsy. Memory was reported to have remained the same for 37.7%, improved for .7%, and worsened for 57.3% (data missing for 4.3%).

TABLE 1. Symptoms Associated with Narcolepsy

Symptom	Troubled moderately or a great deal
Daytime drowsiness	84.5%
Sleep attacks	68.9%
Restless nighttime sleep	61.6%
Vivid imagery on falling asleep	47.7%
Cataplexy	43.2%

TABLE 2. Activities or Experiences that Initiate or Aggravate Symptoms of Narcolepsy

Activity/Experience	Percent
Monotonous activity	62.7%
Reading	59.0%
Too little sleep	58.4%
Boredom	56.4%
Excitement	39.9%
Stress	39.7%

Subjects were given a list of visual problems and asked which ones they had experienced. Subjects reported problems with easy eye fatigue while reading (54.2%), difficulty focusing on objects (44.5%), double vision (31.4%), uncontrolled eyeflickering (26.3%), eyes bothered by fluorescent lights (22.7%), and halos around objects (22.1%).

The lag time between the onset of symptoms of narcolepsy and correct diagnosis was assessed. The mean lag time was 14.63 years (SD = 12.27, range = 0 to 68). In addition, subjects were asked whether they had had difficulty getting appropriate medical care. The majority (56.8%) stated that they had had difficulty.

Social and Economic Domain

Regarding the social and economic aspects of life, subjects were asked how much symptoms of narcolepsy or its treatment had contributed to difficulty with various social aspects of life. Thirty-three percent reported that narcolepsy had contributed moderately or a great deal to social isolation. Narcolepsy also was reported to contribute to difficulty making or keeping friends (18.7%), difficulty with teachers in school (16.0%), and difficulty with classmates or co-workers (14.9%).

Regarding work, the majority (75.2%) reported that narcolepsy had reduced their job performance. Only 10.8% of the sample reported that narcolepsy had *not* reduced their job performance. (Data missing for 14.1%.) Table 3 shows the most frequently reported reasons for problems with jobs. Sleep attacks were the most predominant problem. Subjects also had a great deal of trouble due to problems with concentration and memory. Some subjects experienced personality changes and interpersonal problems due to narcolepsy that were severe enough to cause problems on the job. Subjects were also asked what impact narcolepsy had on their jobs. The most common problem reported was worry about losing their job (33.2%). Some also reported actually losing their jobs (18.6%), as well as losing promotions (16.1%), and receiving decreased wages (10.4%) due to narcolepsy.

TABLE 3. Problems with Jobs

Problem	Percent
Sleep attacks	63.3%
Problems with concentration	40.4%
Problems with memory	32.3%
Personality changes	14.7%
Interpersonal problems	13.7%
Other	11.1%

Psychological/Spiritual Domain

Regarding psychological/spiritual aspects of life, subjects were asked whether they were troubled by recurrent depressed moods. Seventy percent responded that they were troubled by recurrent depressed moods, and 41.2% were troubled either moderately or to a great extent. In addition, self-esteem was assessed by asking subjects how satisfied they were with themselves in general. This was rated on a scale ranging from 1 (very dissatisfied) to 6 (very satisfied). The mean response was 4.34 (SD = 1.40, range = 1 to 6), which indicated that they were only slightly satisfied with themselves.

Family Domain

The final domain focused on family aspects of life. Subjects were asked which symptoms of narcolepsy were most distressing for the people with whom they lived. The symptoms that were reported to be most distressing were sleep attacks and daytime drowsiness. Subjects also were asked if narcolepsy had contributed to difficulties with their family. Respondents stated that narcolepsy had contributed to problems with family members (24.2%) and living partners (24.5%). Narcolepsy was also reported to contribute to difficulties in finding a marital partner/boyfriend/girlfriend (14.9%) and to divorce or separation from spouse (13.9%).

DISCUSSION

The purpose of this study was to assess the quality of life of persons who have narcolepsy. Overall quality of life was evaluated in terms of how satisfied subjects were with the aspects of life that they valued. The narcolepsy group experienced a lower quality of life than did healthy persons. As a group, they were only slightly satisfied with their lives in general.

Health and Functioning

The domain in which subjects reported the lowest quality of life was health and functioning. Respondents were troubled by daytime drowsiness, sleep attacks, restless nighttime sleep, vivid imagery on falling asleep, and cataplexy. The fact that these were problematic was not surprising, since they are classic symptoms of narcolepsy. However, it is disturbing that such large percentages of the group were still troubled by these problems, even though they were being treated medically. The finding that many common activities and experiences, such as reading, excitement, too little sleep, and stress, were reported to bring on symptoms of narcolepsy implies that subjects were required to make major modifications in normal activities of life to attempt to control their symptoms.

Visual problems also interfered with normal functioning. Many of the subjects had trouble with easy eye fatigue while reading, difficulty focusing, double vision, uncontrolled eye flickering, eyes bothered by fluorescent lights, and halos around objects.

A surprising finding was that 57.3% of the sample reported their memory had become worse since developing narcolepsy. Deterioration of memory has not traditionally been recognized as a common problem occurring with narcolepsy. However, these findings demonstrate that loss of memory is a frequent enough problem to warrant serious future study. This issue is discussed in another paper in this volume entitled, "Can We Predict Cognitive Impairment in Narcoleptic Persons?"

Obtaining appropriate treatment for narcolepsy was also a common problem. Respondents reported an unacceptably long lag time between the onset of symptoms of narcolepsy and correct diagnosis and difficulty obtaining appropriate medical care. These findings underscore the need for greater efforts among physicians, teachers, and the general public to make them aware of narcolepsy and better able to recognize it.

Social and Economic Domain

Quality of life was somewhat higher in the social and economic domain. Narcolepsy was found to contribute to social isolation, difficulty making or keeping friends, difficulty with teachers in school, and difficulty with classmates or co-workers. Regarding work, the majority reported that narcolepsy had reduced their job performance. It is disturbing that problems with concentration, memory, and sleep attacks were problematic for so many subjects in the workplace. Thus, even when awake, mental performance was impaired. It is clear from these findings that even though people are being treated for narcolepsy, it is still having a deleterious impact on their work and social lives.

Psychological/Spiritual Domain

Quality of life regarding psychological/spiritual aspects was just slightly higher than that of social and economic aspects, albeit not significantly. Recurrent depressed moods were found to be a major problem for many of the respondents. Forty-one percent were troubled by depression either moderately or to a great extent. These findings concur with those of Broughton et al. (1981), who reported that 51.1% of their sample experienced recurrent depression. Both of these findings were higher than the 28.9% found for a control group (Broughton et al. 1981).

Regarding self-esteem, subjects were only slightly satisfied with themselves. Similarly, Cohen, Ferrans, and Smith report elsewhere in this issue that the self-esteem of persons with narcolepsy was significantly lower than that of the general population, as measured by Rosenberg's Self-Esteem Scale.

Family Domain

The highest quality of life was found in the area of family. Nevertheless, narcolepsy was reported to have contributed to problems with family members, separation and divorce, and difficulty finding a spouse. Sleep attacks and daytime drowsiness were reported to be most distressing to family members.

CONCLUSION

The findings of this study reveal that narcolepsy continues to have a significant negative impact on many aspects of life. The results of this study encourage health care professionals to strive to improve treatment to enhance the quality of life for persons who have narcolepsy. They also reveal the need for greater public and professional awareness of narcolepsy to promote early identification and treatment, as well as greater understanding of the problems faced by persons who have narcolepsy.

REFERENCES

Broughton, R., and Q. Ghanem. 1974. "The Impact of Compound Narcolepsy on the Life of the Patient." In E. Weitzman, C. Guilleminault, W. Dement, and P. Passouant, eds. *Advances in Sleep Research: Narcolepsy.* New York: Spectrum Publications, Inc., pp. 201-220.

Broughton, R., Q. Ghanem, Y. Hishikawa, Y. Sugita, S. Nevsimalova, and B. Roth. 1981. "Life Effects of Narcolepsy in 180 Patients from North America, Asia, and Europe Compared to Matched Controls." *Canadian Journal of Neurological Sciences* 8(4): 299-304.

Broughton, R., Q. Ghanem, Y. Hishikawa, Y. Sugita, S. Nevsimalova, and B. Roth. 1983. "Life Effects of Narcolepsy: Relationships to Geographic Origin (North American, Asian or European) and to Other Patient and Illness Variables." *Canadian Journal of Neurological Sciences* 10:100-104.

Broughton, R., A. Guberman, and J. Roberts. 1984. "Comparison of the Psychosocial Effects of Epilepsy and Narcolepsy/Cataplexy: A Controlled Study." *Epilepsia* 25(4): 423-433.

Ferrans, C. 1990. "Development of a Quality of Life Index for Patients with Cancer." *Oncology Nursing Forum* 17(3) suppl:15-19.

Ferrans, C. and M. Powers. 1985. "Quality of Life Index: Development and Psychometric Properties." *Advances in Nursing Science* 8(1): 15-24.

Psychosocial Impact
of Narcolepsy-Cataplexy

Roger J. Broughton

Questionnaire studies comparing patients with narcolepsy-cataplexy to age- and sex-matched controls have shown that narcolepsy has a very significant psychosocial impact (Broughton et al. 1981). Narcoleptics attribute these problems directly to their condition and, more particularly, to the persistent excessive daytime sleepiness rather than to the brief episodic attacks of sleep, cataplexy, or other symptoms.

In this study of 180 narcoleptics, subjects were found to have a high frequency of reduced job performance, fear of job loss, reduced earnings, prevention of promotions, actual job loss, and disability status. Although they achieved educational levels equal to those of controls, they more frequently believed that their condition led to poor marks, suffered interpersonal problems with teachers, or had embarrassment due to symptoms. The narcoleptics had a very high frequency of falling asleep at the wheel while driving, more frequent near accidents while driving, more actual driving accidents, higher automobile insurance rates, and higher incidence of suspended driving license. They also had more frequent household and occupational accidents, with a high frequency of accidents related to smoking. Narcoleptics had problems planning recreation; interpersonal problems at work, school, and home; and they suffered from a variety of symptoms reducing quality of life, including recurrent depression, memory problems, sensitivity to alcohol, re-

Roger J. Broughton, MD, PhD, ACP, is Director, Division of Neurology, Department of Medicine, Sleep Disorders Center, Ottawa General Hospital, Canada.

duced sexual drive, and (in males) more frequent impotence than controls.

The psychosocial effects were essentially identical between similar populations from North America, Japan, and Czechoslovakia, indicating that the effects are an integral part of the disease and are similar whatever the genetic origin or cultural experience of the person afflicted (Broughton et al. 1983).

Memory problems in narcoleptics are common and were studied by objective psychological memory tests. Patients were chosen who were subjectively judged to have great problems. But in the laboratory we found them to perform as well as normal subjects whether on or off medication. It appears that narcoleptics have an ability to "rally" and overcome their pathological drowsiness for at least short periods of time in a laboratory setting (Aguirre et al. 1985). These negative results do not indicate that no memory deficits are present in narcolepsy, but rather that they are entirely attributable to drowsiness and so are potentially reversible, rather than representing permanent effects.

Comparisons of narcolepsy-cataplexy with the condition of idiopathic central nervous system (CNS) hypersomnia (characterized by long and deep night sleep, long daytime sleep episodes, and excessive daytime sleepiness) showed that the two clinical conditions are very similar in respect to psychosocial effects. The main differences were for situations in which the more imperative and overwhelming nature of sleep attacks in narcolepsy played a role, such as in household and smoking accidents, driving problems, and impact on recreational activities (Broughton et al. 1980).

Narcolepsy-cataplexy has also been compared to epilepsy, another chronic neurological condition characterized by episodic symptoms (seizures), for which a large literature on psychosocial effects exists. We found that narcoleptics were even more impaired than epileptics in all of their psychosocial parameters other than education (a specific learning disability exists in temporal lobe epileptics, a major group in the patient population), and ability to hold a driver's license (specific regulations exist for epilepsy) (Broughton et al. 1984). This difference between conditions appeared to be due to the chronic and unrelenting excessive daytime sleepiness which characterizes narcolepsy, whereas epileptics are relatively asymptomatic between attacks.

There is much need for counseling narcoleptics concerning the psychosocial impact so that they can optimize adaptation to their disease and be realistic in their expectations. In situations in which work problems are particularly marked, it is often also helpful to involve the employer. Once a narcoleptic person has "gone public," the psychosocial problems with employers, friends, druggists, and others generally decrease. It is unfortunate that the medical treatment of excessive daytime sleepiness in narcolepsy-cataplexy is still so inadequate, in as much as this is the symptom which causes most of the psychosocial impact.

REFERENCES

Aguirre, M., R. Broughton, and D. Stuss. 1985. "Does Memory Dysfunction Exist in Narcolepsy-Cataplexy?" *Journal of Clinical Experiments in Neuropsychology* 7:14-24.

Broughton, R., Q. Ghanem, Y. Hishikawa, Y. Sugita, S. Nevsimalova, and B. Roth. 1981. "Life Effects of Narcolepsy in 180 Patients from North America, Asia and Europe Compared to Matched Controls." *Canadian Journal of Neurological Science* 8:299-304.

Broughton, R., Q. Ghanem, Y. Hishikawa, Y. Sugita, S. Nevsimalova, and B. Roth. 1983. "Life Effects of Narcolepsy: Relationships to Geographic Origin (North American, Asian or European) and to Other Patient and Illness Variables." *Canadian Journal of Neurological Science* 10:100-104.

Broughton, R., A. Guberman, and J. Roberts. 1984. "Comparison of the Psychosocial Effects of Epilepsy and Narcolepsy-Cataplexy." *Epilepsia* 25(4):423-433.

Broughton, R., S. Nevsimalova, and B. Roth. 1980. "The Socioeconomic Effects of Ideopathic Hypersomnia: Comparison with Controls and with Compound Narcoleptics." In L. Popoviciu, B. Asgian and G. Badin, eds. *Sleep 1978.* Basel: Karger, pp. 103-111.

Psychosocial Impact of Narcolepsy-Cataplexy with Comparisons to Idiopathic Hypersomnia and Epilepsy

Roger J. Broughton

This paper summarizes a series of studies on the psychosocial aspects of narcolepsy completed over the past 15 years. At the time of beginning these studies, apart from a report on driving in narcoleptics by Bartels and Kusakcioglu (1985), which involved a mixed group of abnormally sleepy patients including narcoleptics, no other publications on the topic had been published. This was despite widespread clinical experience of the often devastating impact of narcolepsy on work, education, recreation, accidents, interpersonal relationships, and other parameters of quality of life.

Roger J. Broughton, MD, PhD, ACP, is Director, Division of Neurology, Department of Medicine, Sleep Disorders Center Ottawa General Hospital, Canada.

The author thanks the following who participated in the collaborative studies mentioned: Qais Ghanem, currently in St. Catharines, Canada; Alan Guberman, Division of Neurology, University of Ottawa, Ottawa, Canada; Yasuo Hishikawa, Department of Neuropsychiatry, Akita University, Akita, Japan; Sonya Nevsimalova, Neurology Clinic, Charles University, Prague, Czechoslovakia; the late Bedrich Roth, Neurology Clinic, Charles University, Prague, Czechoslovakia; Yashiro Sugita, Department of Neuropsychiatry, Osaka University, Osaka, Japan.

The author acknowledges financial support by the Medical Council of Canada for all five studies, and thanks Mrs. Barbara Reynolds for her secretarial support.

37

PSYCHOSOCIAL EFFECTS OF NARCOLEPSY

After an initial preliminary report based exclusively upon North American patients (Broughton and Ghanem 1976) a three-center international study involving patients in Ottawa, Prague, and Osaka was launched. It surveyed 60 patients and age- and sex-matched normal controls in each of the participating centers using a comprehensive questionnaire (Broughton et al. 1981). Questionnaires were translated from English into Japanese, Czech, and Slovak, and were completed with close physician monitoring. Our main objectives were to do a broad survey of psychosocial aspects and to determine whether or not the impact was due to the intermittent tetrad of diagnostic symptoms (especially sleep attacks and cataplexy) or to the daytime sleepiness persistent between the episodic symptoms.

Among the many statistically significant findings were:

a. *Work* — Narcoleptics more frequently had reduced performance (78% in narcoleptics), fear of job loss (49%), reduced earnings (47%), prevention of promotions (38%), actual job loss (21%), and disability status (11%).

b. *Education* — Although narcoleptics achieved equal educational levels, they more frequently believed their condition led to poor marks (51%), or suffered from interpersonal problems with teachers (34%) and embarrassment (32%).

c. *Driving* — Narcoleptics had more frequently fallen asleep driving (67%), more frequent near accidents (67%), more frequent actual accidents (37%), higher insurance rates (16%) and greater frequency of suspended license (6%).

d. *Accidents* — Narcoleptics had much more frequent household and occupational accidents (49%), and more frequent accidents attributable to smoking (also 49%).

e. *Recreation* — Narcoleptics had frequent sleep attacks during recreational activities and had more problems in planning recreation (27%).

f. *Interpersonal relationships* — Interpersonal problems at work, school, and home were much more frequent in narcoleptics. They often (34%) believed that others were intolerant of their symptoms, and many had problems filling prescriptions.

g. *Symptoms* — A number of nondiagnostic symptoms that reduced quality of life were more frequent in narcoleptics. These included: imbalance (56%); recurrent depression (51%); memory problems (49%), mainly (81% of those affected) for recent events; marked sensitivity to alcohol (32%); reduced sexual drive (17% of both sexes); and impotence (15% of males).

These summary statistics quantified the impact of the disease. But it was the individual forms that documented and elaborated on particular life experiences. These were often extremely disheartening. There were persons whose marriages had broken up due to the disease. Some had suffered terrible accidents or burns. A number of patients had had their cataplexy induced by others for "fun." A novelist lost his only manuscript copy of a book on a bus during an episode of behavioral automatism.

Concerning the mechanism of these life effects, a checklist was provided for possible causes of problems related to work, education, driving and accidents. It revealed that the most common factor was excessive daytime sleepiness, rather than the episodic diagnostic narcolepsy symptoms or other possible causes.

COMPARISON OF EFFECTS BY GEOGRAPHIC ORIGIN

In order to determine if the life-effects varied according to geographic origin, whether by cultural or genetic factors, a comparison was made between life-effects of patients (N = 60 each) from each of the North American, Japanese, and Czechoslovakian subgroups for each of the parameters (Broughton et al. 1983). The main finding of this data reanalysis was that there were, in fact, very few differences for any of the 160 items sampled. This supported the belief that the main socioeconomic effects are an *integral* part of the disease and are similar whatever the genetic origin or cultural experience of the person afflicted.

The few differences that emerged were explicable mainly by cultural differences. Thoughts of suicide were more common in the Japanese patients, whose culture has a greater tradition of using suicide as a "way out." Driving and driving accidents were significantly less frequent in Czechoslovaks, whose culture has longstanding severe restrictions and penalties for driving by narcoleptics. And smoking accidents were less common in the Japanese, who have a lower frequency of smoking.

MEMORY PROBLEMS IN NARCOLEPSY

It had been found, as mentioned, that subjective memory problems are particularly common in narcoleptics. Patients frequently keep long lists and use other strategies for short-term recall. These subjective problems were investigated using a neuropsychological test battery involving various measures, which sampled immediate, short-term, and long-term memory and employed both auditory and visual modes of presentation. Narcoleptics were selected who complained of marked sleepiness. They were assessed both on and off treatment and were compared to a matched group of normal controls. This study was done in collaboration with neuropsychologist colleagues Marisa Aguirre and Donald Stuss (Aguirre et al. 1985).

The unexpected finding of this study was that there were no significant differences in memory function for any of the parameters employed. This negative result appeared entirely due to the ability of narcoleptics to rally for short periods of time and perform at normal or near normal levels. This had been previously shown for a number of other performance tests in untreated narcoleptics by Valley and Broughton (1981, 1983). It was only in the very boring, and particularly the very prolonged, tests that narcoleptics did poorly. During short challenging tasks, including memory tests, they appear to be able to rally and sustain alertness.

COMPARISON WITH IDIOPATHIC CNS HYPERSOMNIA

Because most of the impact of the disease appeared due to sleepiness, it was decided to compare persons with narcolepsy-cataplexy syndrome to those with a diagnosis of idiopathic central nervous system (CNS) hypersomnia (Broughton et al. 1980). In the latter condition, cataplexy, sleep paralysis, vivid hypnagogic hallucinations, and other expressions of abnormal REM sleep do not occur. Idiopathic CNS hypersomnia is a relatively rare condition, so that only 30 patients in each group were compared. The questionnaire was identical to that of the original studies.

It was found that the idiopathic hypersomniacs had similar, and sometimes greater, problems than those of narcoleptics. This is perhaps due to the even greater pressure for sleep and greatly increased amounts of sleep during the 24 hours characteristic of this condition. Narcoleptics, however, suffered higher impairment in those situations in which the more paroxysmal and imperative nature of their symptoms (particularly sleep attacks and cataplexy) played a role, such as in household and smoking accidents, driving problems, and recreational activities. The overall similar nature of the impact supported again the belief that it is the chronic, unrelenting daytime sleepiness (experienced by both groups) which is the major cause of the psychosocial problems.

COMPARISON WITH EPILEPSY

A more recent study of the psychosocial effects of narcolepsy involved comparison with matched patients with epilepsy (Broughton et al. 1984). Epilepsy was chosen for comparison, because it also is a chronic neurological condition with paroxysmal attacks. Moreover, there is a very extensive literature on the psychosocial aspects of epilepsy. In order to have a reasonably comparable group, epileptics were excluded who had severe organic brain disease. All of the epileptic patients retained in this comparison had either primary generalized epilepsy or complex partial seizures of temporal lobe origin, but always without significant brain lesions on CT scan, NMR or other neuroradiological procedures.

This study confirmed the already well-documented deleterious effects of epilepsy upon work, education, occupational and household accidents, recreation, personality, interpersonal relationships, and other parameters mentioned. However, the narcoleptics were either equally or more impaired on virtually all parameters. Specifically, narcoleptics showed greater frequencies than epileptics of disease-attributed reduced performance at work, poorer driving records, higher accident rates from smoking, greater problems in planning recreation, and deficits on a large number of other significant parameters. The only parameters where the reverse was true involved educational problems and ability to maintain a driving license, which were more impacted by epilepsy. The great problems with learning and education are already well-documented in epileptics, particularly for temporal lobe epilepsy. The difference in ability to maintain a driving license is explicable by the more stringent regulations excluding driving for that condition.

The greater overall psychosocial impact of narcolepsy appeared to be due to the fact that persons with such forms of epilepsy are relatively normal between the intermittent seizures, whereas the narcoleptics suffered from chronic sleepiness between episodic symptoms.

CONCLUSION

It now appears well-documented from these studies, and from those of other centers, that narcolepsy indeed has a very significant psychosocial impact. That most of these problems are due to excessive daytime sleepiness, and that it is the sleepiness which is the most refractory symptom to treatment (Guilleminault and Dement 1974; Broughton and Mamelak 1979), make it doubly imperative that the problem of pathological sleepiness be better understood and that improvements in its therapy be achieved.

REFERENCES

Aguirre, M., R. Broughton, and D. Stuss. 1985. "Does Memory Dysfunction Exist in Narcolepsy-Cataplexy?" *Journal of Clinical Experiments in Neuropsychology* 7:14-24.

Bartels, E. C. and O. Kusakcioglu, 1965. "Narcolepsy: A Possible Cause of Automobile Accidents," *Lahey Clinical Foundation Bulletin* 14: 22-26.

Broughton, R. and Q. Ghanem. 1976. "The Impact of Compound Narcolepsy on the Life of the Patient." In C. Guilleminault, W. C. Dement and P. Passouant, eds. *Narcolepsy.* New York: Spectrum, pp. 659-666.

Broughton, R. and M. Mamelak. 1979. "The Treatment of Narcolepsy-Cataplexy with Nocturnal Gamma-Hydroxybutyrate." *Canadian Journal of Neurological Sciences* 6:1-6.

Broughton, R., Q. Ghanem, Y. Hishikawa, Y. Sugita, S. Nevsimalova, and B. Roth. 1981. "Life Effects of Narcolepsy in 180 Patients from North America, Asia and Europe Compared to Matched Controls." *Canadian Journal of Neurological Sciences* 8:299-304.

Broughton, R., Q. Ghanem, Y. Hishikawa, Y. Sugita, S. Nevsimalova, and B. Roth. 1983. "Life Effects of Narcolepsy: Relationships to Geographic Origin (North American, Asian or European) and to Other Patient and Illness Variables." *Canadian Journal of Neurological Sciences* 10:100-104.

Broughton, R., S. Nevsimalova, and B. Roth. 1980. "The Socioeconomic Effects of Idiopathic Hypersomnia: Comparison with Controls and with Compound Narcoleptics." In. L. Popoviciu, B. Asgian, and G. Badiu, eds. *Sleep 1978*. Basel: Karger, pp. 103-111.

Broughton, R., A. Guberman, and J. Roberts. 1984. "Comparison of Psychosocial Effects of Epilepsy and of Narcolepsy-Cataplexy: A Controlled Study." *Epilepsia* 57:303-309.

Guilleminault, C. and W. C. Dement. 1974. "Pathologies of Excessive Sleep." In E. Weitzman, ed. *Advances in Sleep Research*. New York: Spectrum, pp. 345-390.

Valley, V. and R. Broughton. 1981. "Daytime Performances Deficits and Physiological Vigilance in Untreated Patients with Narcolepsy-Cataplexy Compared to Controls." *Review of EEG Neurophysiology (Paris)* 11:133-139.

Valley, V. and R. Broughton. 1983. "The Physiological (EEG) Nature of Drowsiness and its Relation to Performance Deficits in Narcoleptics." *Electroencephalograph Clinical Neurophysiology* 55:243-251.

Self-Esteem in Persons with Narcolepsy

Felissa L. Cohen
Carol E. Ferrans
Karen M. Smith

Self-concept and self-esteem are terms that in the past have been used widely and sometimes loosely in the literature. Part of the explanation for this has to do with the wide range of theoretical perspectives bearing on these terms and the variety of measurement orientations. More recently, there has been some agreement on the definition and measurement. In general, self-concept can be thought of in a cognitive aspect. It reflects a total or overall appraisal of the self that can be global or specific. It is not merely how one feels about oneself but how one feels about how one *sees* oneself. It is an evaluation of self-worth (Stanwyck 1983; Breytspraak and George 1982).

The purposes of this study were:

1. To examine self-esteem in persons with narcolepsy,
2. To ascertain the relationship between various demographic and other variables and self-esteem in persons with narcolepsy and

Felissa L. Cohen, RN, PhD, FAAN, is Director, Center for Narcolepsy Research, and Professor of Medical/Surgical Nursing, College of Nursing, University of Illinois at Chicago, Chicago, IL. Carol E. Ferrans, RN, PhD, is affiliated with the College of Nursing, University of Illinois at Chicago, Chicago, IL. Karen M. Smith, PhD, is Senior Research Specialist, Center for Narcolepsy Research, College of Nursing, University of Illinois at Chicago, Chicago, IL.

This research was supported in part by Mr. J. A. Piscopo, founder and retired Chairman of the Board of Directors of Pansophic Systems, Inc. The authors would like to thank the American Narcolepsy Association for its assistance with the data collection for this study.

3. To compare self-esteem in persons with narcolepsy and the general population.

A search of the literature revealed many studies on self-esteem in a variety of chronic illnesses and conditions but none were found that examined self-esteem in persons who had narcolepsy. The wealth of literature dealing with self-esteem in a variety of other states and conditions is beyond the scope of this paper.

METHODS

Participants in this study consisted of respondents to a mailed questionnaire that was distributed under the auspices of the Center for Narcolepsy Research. The methodology employed in this study is reported in the paper entitled "The Quality of Life of Persons with Narcolepsy" that appears elsewhere in this volume.

The Rosenberg Self-Esteem Scale was used to measure self-esteem. This instrument consists of 10 items reported along a 4-point continuum from strongly agree to strongly disagree. Higher scores indicate higher self-esteem (Breytspraak and George 1982; Rosenberg 1965). Various formal studies of reliability have ranged from a reproducibility coefficient of 0.92, to a test-retest correlation of 0.85, to an internal consistency rating of 0.74. Formal tests of validity demonstrate good discriminant validity in addition to concurrent and construct validity (Breytspraak and George 1982).

As discussed in other papers in this volume, self-esteem was part of a questionnaire packet sent to random samples of persons with narcolepsy and the general population. The latter was represented by selection from the phone book in the town of Rockford, Illinois. The final sample size for the self-esteem segment for persons with narcolepsy was 485. Demographic information and other data relating to aspects of self-described severity of illness were also collected. Characteristics of the final sample are shown in Table 1.

RESULTS

For persons with narcolepsy, scores on the Rosenberg Self-Esteem Scale actually ranged from 18 to 40 with a mean of 30.18 (s.d. = 6.11).

Subjects were asked to rate their perceived symptom severity. The possible categories ranged from mild through extremely severe. Subjects reported these as follows: 23.1% mild, 41.9% moderate, 27.2% severe, and 7.8% extremely severe. Mean scores for self-esteem using the Rosenberg scale were calculated for each grouping of symptom severity. These data are shown in Table 2. Not surprisingly, those with mild symptoms had self-esteem scores that were significantly higher than all other categories [$F(3,476) = 19.65$, $p < .0001$, Tukey post hoc test comparison $p < .05$]. An analysis of variance yielded significant differences between the severity groups [$F(3,476) = 19.65$, $p < .001$], Tukey post hoc comparisons showed that those with the mild or moderate symptoms have significantly higher self-esteem than those with severe or extremely severe symptoms ($p < .05$).

Persons with narcolepsy were also asked whether they evidenced a variety of possible symptoms of narcolepsy. Symptoms that are typically considered to be part of the narcoleptic tetrad—excessive daytime sleepiness, hypnagogic hallucinations, cataplexy, and sleep paralysis—were scored. Scores were grouped by severity. Group 1 was the least severe and group 4 was the most severe. Statistically significant differences were noted among the self-esteem means for these groups. Those with the least severe classic symptomatology had the highest self-esteem, while those with the most severe had the lowest self-esteem [$F(3, 429) = 21.96$, $p < .001$]. These data were consistent with the self-classification of the respondents.

The important area of employment was next. Self-esteem scores of narcoleptic respondents were examined in relation to employment status. Those persons who were students, employed full-time, or retired had the highest self-esteem scores, while those who were unemployed or who considered themselves disabled had the lowest self-esteem scores. These differences were statistically significant [$F(6, 477) = 9.92$, $p < .001$]. When asked to what extent job performance was affected by narcolepsy, those who perceived the least reduction in job performance had the highest self-esteem scores [$F(3, 419) = 31.18$, $p < .001$]. Tukey post hoc comparisons found no difference between those who perceived no reduction or slight reduction of performance in their self-esteem ratings ($p > .05$).

The level of educational attainment was also examined. Those

TABLE 1. Descriptive Statistics for Respondents to Self-Esteem Study in Percent (n = 489)[a]

Variable	N	%
Age		
18-40	98	18.2
41-55	200	37.1
56-65	153	28.4
66 & older	83	15.4
Sex		
Male	211	43.5
Female	272	56.36
Ethnicity		
American Indian	8	1.6
Black	14	2.9
White	456	94.0
Oriental	1	.2
Spanish American	2	.4
Marital Status		
Single	32	7.6
Married	334	68.9
Widowed	31	6.4
Separated/ Divorced	81	16.8

[a]Totals vary due to nonresponses

persons with narcolepsy who had the highest educational attainment had significantly higher self-esteem than those with lower achievement [$F(4, 479) = 5.16$, $p < .001$]. Those who did not graduate from high school had significantly lower self-esteem than those who had some college level education or higher.

Variable	N	%
Work Status		
Employed Full Time	205	42.3
Employed Part time	60	12.4
Housewife	51	10.5
Student	7	1.4
Unemployed	19	3.9
Disabled	46	9.5
Retired	96	19.8

Years of Work Experience		
Less than 1 year	3	.6
1-9 years	31	5.8
10-19 years	69	12.8
20-29 years	104	19.3
30 years or more	215	39.9

TABLE 2. Self-Esteem and Self-Reported Severity[a] in Narcoleptic Subjects

Symptom Severity	Self-Esteem	
	Mean	S.D.
Mild	33.0	5.7
Moderate	30.6	5.2
Severe	28.2	6.4
Extremely Severe	26.2	6.7

[a]$[F(3, 476) = 19.65, p < .0001]$

How others appraise a person is a component of that person's self-esteem. Respondents were asked how understanding about narcolepsy they believed their spouse or significant other to be. There were statistically significant differences among those ratings in regard to self-esteem means [F(3, 456) = 5.92, p < .001]. In general, those who rated their spouses as more understanding had higher self-esteem ratings. Slight differences in understanding were not significantly different. For example, there were no statistically significant differences between those who rated their spouse as showing no understanding and those who rated them as showing slight understanding (p > .05). Those spouses who were perceived as moderately understanding and those who were very understanding showed no statistically significant difference when a Tukey's test was applied (p > .05).

Perceived understanding regarding narcolepsy of those persons who were not significant others was also examined. These were rated as not at all, slightly, moderately, or very understanding. The self-esteem means were compared by perceived level of understanding. The greater the perceived understanding of others, the higher the respondents' self-esteem [F(3, 475 = 23.41, p < .001]. Tukey posthoc analysis indicated that those who viewed other people as either being not at all understanding or slightly understanding of their symptoms had significantly lower self-esteem than respondents who viewed others as being moderately or very understanding (p < .05).

Persons with narcolepsy were also asked the extent to which they believed their symptoms contributed to problems with others. Those who believed that their symptoms contributed greatly to such problems had the lowest self-esteem, and these differences were again statistically significant [F(3, 456) = 9.64, p < .001). Tukey post hoc comparisons found that those who thought people were very understanding of their symptoms had significantly higher self-esteem than those who rated the degree of people's understanding as moderate, slight, or not at all. Those who thought people were moderately understanding of their symptoms had significantly higher self-esteem than those who felt people were not understanding at all (p < .05).

The demographic variables of age and gender in narcoleptics were examined in respect to self-esteem scores. There were no statistically significant differences in self-esteem scores between males and females although males have shown higher self-esteem scores in other studies (Durham and Cohen 1990). Likewise, in regard to age, there were no statistically significant differences among subjects of different ages when examined in 10-year intervals.

Finally, the self-esteem scores of persons with narcolepsy and persons in the general population were compared. There were statistically significant differences. For persons with narcolepsy, mean self-esteem scores were 30.18 (s.d. = 6.11). Not surprisingly, the self-esteem means were higher for those in the general population. The mean self-esteem score for the general sample was 32.91 (s.d. = 4.66). These two means were found to be statistically significantly different [$t(804) = 6.80, p < .001$]. Interestingly, when looking at the overall means, those narcoleptics with mild symptoms, less perceived job problems, and higher perceived understanding of others (spouse/significant other or more distant others) had self-esteem means that were similar to the general population means.

In summary, self-esteem in this sample of narcoleptics was not related to biological variables such as age and sex. Those variables that were important were symptom severity, perceived understanding of their spouses, perceived understanding of other people, employment, perception of the influence of symptoms on job performance, and educational achievement. Some of these variables are less susceptible to manipulation. Others, however, could be responsive to various approaches, leading to more positive feelings about self.

REFERENCES

Breytspraak, L. M. and L. K. George. 1981. "Self-Concept and Self-Esteem." In D. J. Mangta and W. A. Peterson, eds. *Research Instruments in Social Gerontology*. Minneapolis, MN: University of Minnesota Press, pp. 241-302.

Durham, J. D. and F. L. Cohen. 1990. "Men in Nursing: Who Wants Them, Who Needs Them?" Paper presented at the 13th Conference of the Southeast Clinical Specialist in Psychiatric Nursing. Gatlinburg, TN, September 6, 1990.

Rosenberg, M. 1965. *Society and the Adolescent Self-Image*. Princeton, NJ: Princeton University Press.

Stanwyck, D. J. 1983. "Self-esteem Through the Life Span." *Family Community Health* 6(2):11-28.

Depressive Symptomatology in Narcolepsy

Sharon L. Merritt
Felissa L. Cohen
Karen M. Smith

People with narcolepsy report experiencing a wide variety of symptoms associated with this disease, including depression. Most researchers have concentrated their attention on trying to understand the pathophysiologic mechanisms underlying the symptoms rather than how the symptoms of this disorder may be related to more general mental states like depression (Broughton and Ghanem 1976). Irrespective of cause, the intensity of depressive symptoms can vary. The presence of symptoms does not necessarily indicate that a person with a depressed mood would be diagnosed in the psychiatric sense as being clinically depressed. However, significant depressive symptoms may mean the quality of life of people with narcolepsy is compromised. The purposes of this research were to determine the prevalence of depressive symptoms among a national sample of people with narcolepsy and to determine if the intensity of depressive symptoms being experienced was influenced

Sharon L. Merritt, RN, EdD, is Assistant Director, Center for Narcolepsy Research, College of Nursing, University of Illinois at Chicago, Chicago, IL. Felissa L. Cohen, RN, PhD, FAAN, is Director, Center for Narcolepsy Research, and Professor of Medical/Surgical Nursing, College of Nursing, University of Illinois at Chicago, Chicago, IL. Karen M. Smith, PhD, is Senior Research Specialist, Center for Narcolepsy Research, College of Nursing, University of Illinois at Chicago, Chicago, IL.

This research was supported in part by Mr. J. A. Piscopo, founder and retired Chairman of the Board of Directors of Pansophic Systems, Inc. The authors wish to thank the American Narcolepsy Association for its assistance in carrying out this research.

53

by personal characteristics and the presence of other narcolepsy-related symptoms.

BACKGROUND

Studies using self-report as well as traditional psychiatric measures have found significant depression among narcoleptics. People newly diagnosed with narcolepsy have reported that depression was the personality change they noted at disease onset (Broughton and Ghanem 1976). Recurrent episodes of depression have been reported by 51% of people with narcolepsy (Broughton, Guberman, and Roberts 1984). When compared to matched normal controls and/or people with sleep apnea, people with narcolepsy have demonstrated social withdrawal and a greater depressed mood (Beutler et al. 1981). McMahon et al. (1982), based on their findings of low levels of emotional security and social interaction among people with narcolepsy, suggested that further research was needed to determine if the emotional effects arise from the disorder, from the attitudes of narcoleptics about the disease, or from the behavior of others toward people with narcolepsy.

METHODS

Design and Instrument

Seven hundred people with narcolepsy (response rate = 61.4%) participated in this retrospective descriptive study. Subjects were chosen randomly from the patient rolls of the American Narcolepsy Association (ANA) to anonymously and voluntarily complete a mailed five-part, self-administering instrument, the Narcolepsy Information Questionnaire (NIQ). This report focuses on data obtained from Parts I and V of the NIQ. Information from data obtained with other parts of the NIQ can be found in other chapters in this volume.

Part I provided information about the usual demographic characteristics of the sample as well as experiences with a comprehensive list of narcolepsy symptoms. Each item (symptom) is rated from 0-3 (0 = never experience to 3 = experience 3/4 of the time or more). Scores for symptom categories and their derivation are presented in Figure 1. Part V consisted of the Center for Epidemiologic Studies Depression Scale (CES-D). This instrument contains 20 items that were selected to study the prevalence of depressive symptoms in the general population. Each item is rated according to how many days within the past week a respondent has experienced the symptom (0 = less than 1 day to 3 = experienced 5-7 days). Scores are obtained by summing the item ratings and range from 0 to 60. A cut-off score of 16 or above indicates the presence of significant depressive symptomatology. Internal consistency has been found to be about 0.85 with stability (test-retest) correlations of about 0.5.

FIGURE 1. Derivation of Narcolepsy Symptom Scores

Symptom Scores	Symptoms
Classic Score (sum of 4 itmes * 10)	Sleep attacks, cataplexy, sleep paralysis, hypnagogic hallucinations
New Classic (1 item * 10 plys classic score	Classic score plus nighttime sleeping difficulties
Associate Score (sum of 3 items * 10)	Automatic behavior, snoring, nightmares
Other Score (sum of 3 items * 10)	Sleepwalking, muscle spasms, visual disturbances
Learning/Memory Score (sum of 4 items * 10)	Difficulty concentrating, learning problems, forgetfulness, memory problems
Total Score	Sum of classic, associated, other, learning/memory scores and new classic item

Sample

The sample for this portion of the NIQ analysis consisted of 631 respondents 18 years of age or older with nonmissing CES-D data. The most frequent age category was 41-55 years of age (34% of the respondents). The majority of subjects were white (93.51%), female (61.17%), married (63.8%), high school graduates (33%), employed at least part-time (51.2%), and had an income of $19,999 or less a year (54%).

FINDINGS AND DISCUSSION

Pharmacologic Treatment

People with narcolepsy are often treated with drugs that could have an effect on depressive symptoms. One-way analysis of variance revealed that there were no significant differences in mean CES-D scores between subjects in five different drug categories [F (df 626, 4) $= .249$, $p < .911$]. The pharmacologic treatment of respondents was not a factor that affected depressive symptomatology findings.

CES-D Scores

About 49% (N = 308) of the respondents scored at or above the cut-off score of 16, indicating a high proportion of the narcoleptic respondents were experiencing depressive symptoms. The proportion of subjects in the general population scoring above 15 has been found to be from 9-31% (Boyd and Weissman 1982; Eaton and Kessler 1981). The proportion of the narcoleptic sample experiencing depression is substantially above what has been found in the general population.

Personal Characteristics and Depressive Symptoms

Chi-square analyses were performed to determine what proportion of subjects in the various categories of personal characteristics scored at or above the cut-off score of 16. The proportion of subjects scoring significantly differently on the CES-D were as follows:

1. *Age* — younger subjects (18-40) experienced significantly more depressive symptoms, $X^2 = 9.632$, p < .02;
2. *Marital status* — married subjects had significantly *lower* CES-D scores, $X^2 = 22.54$, p < .0002;
3. *Education* — narcoleptics with less education tended to experience more symptoms, $X^2 = 10.614$, p < .02;
4. *Income* — subjects at lower income levels had significantly higher CES-D scores, $X^2 = 11.614$, p < .02.

These findings are somewhat similar to those of national samples of the general population. Eaton and Kessler (1981) found significantly higher rates of depression among younger people and persons with lower incomes. Radloff and Locke (1986) reported similar findings among black subjects in the general population.

Depressive Symptomatology and Narcolepsy Symptoms

T-tests for independent samples were used to determine if respondents with a CES-D score of 16 or greater reported experiencing narcolepsy symptoms more frequently than narcoleptic subjects in the 15 or below CES-D group (see Figure 2). Narcoleptic respondents with high CES-D scores (16 or greater) had significantly higher (p. < .05) symptom scale scores in all of the symptom categories. Mean score differences ranged from a low of about 6 for the associated symptoms to a high of about 21 for the learning and memory symptoms.

CONCLUSION

The people with narcolepsy who completed the CES-D in this study demonstrated a higher prevalence of depressive symptomatology than has been found in the general population. In terms of demographic characteristics, the prevalence of depressive symptoms seems to follow a pattern that is similar to what has been demonstrated in the general population. Additionally, the narcoleptic respondents with CES-D scores at or above 16 report experiencing

FIGURE 2. Mean Symptom Scores by CES Group

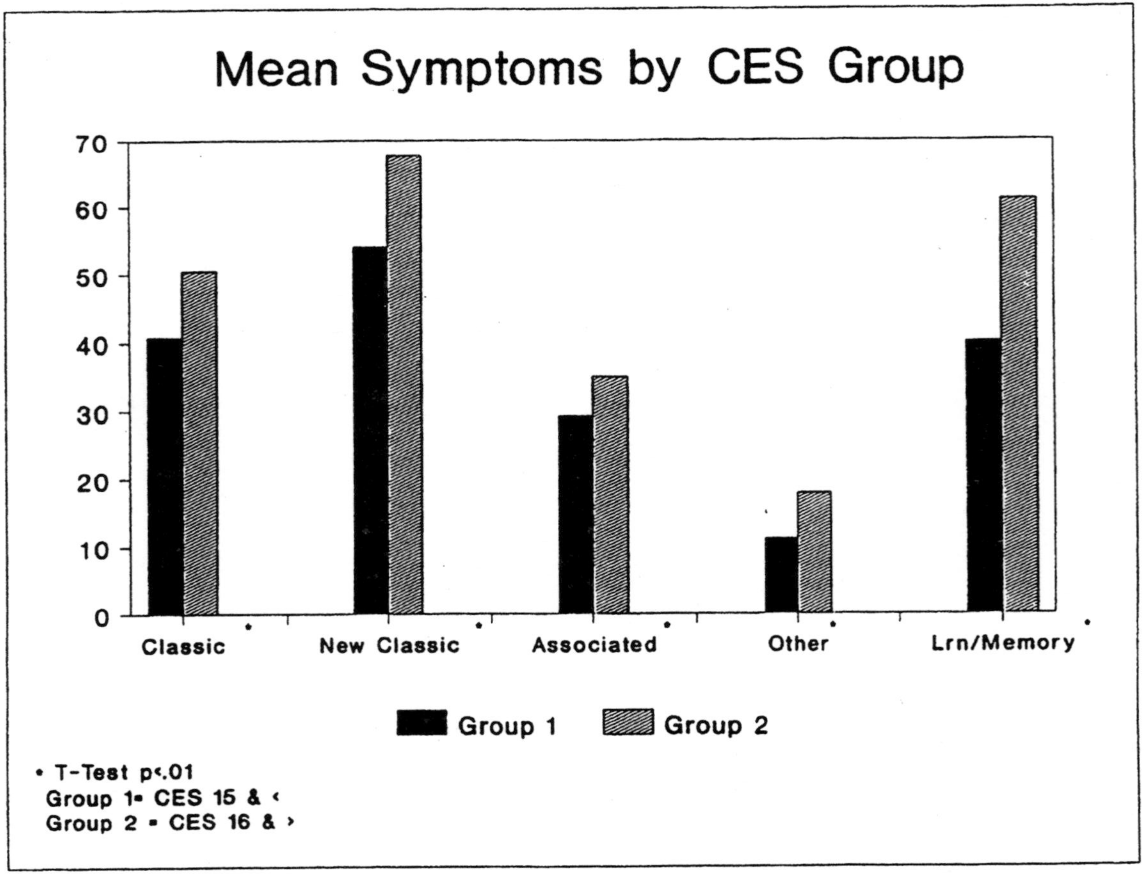

58

significantly more symptoms of narcolepsy across all of the symptom categories. The prevalence of depressive symptoms among this sample suggests that health care professionals need to be more sensitive to screening for and treating these symptoms among people with narcolepsy. Depressive symptoms may add significant burden and interfere with the quality of life above and beyond the disease-specific symptoms associated with this disorder.

REFERENCES

Beutler, L. E., J. C. Ware, I. Karacan, and J. I. Thornby. 1981. "Differentiating Psychological Characteristics of Patients With Sleep Apnea and Narcolepsy." *Sleep* 4: 39-47.

Boyd, J. H., and M. M. Weissman. 1982. "The Epidemiology of Affective Disorders: Depressive Symptoms, Nonbipolar Depression, and Bipolar Disorder." In E. S. Paykel, ed. *Handbook of Affective Disorders*. New York: Churchill Livingstone, pp. 109-125.

Broughton, R., and Q. Ghanem. 1976. "The Impact of Compound Narcolepsy on the Life of the Patient." In C. Gulleminault, W. C Dement, and P. Passouant, eds. *Narcolepsy: Advances in Sleep Research*, vol. 3. New York: Spectrum, pp. 201-219.

Broughton, R., A. Guberman, and J. Roberts. 1984. "Comparison of the Psychosocial Effects of Epilepsy and Narcolepsy/Cataplexy: A Controlled Study." *Epilesia* 25: 423-432.

Eaton, W. W., and L. G. Kessler. 1981. "Rates of Symptoms of Depression in a National Sample." *American Journal of Epidemiology* 114: 528-538.

McMahon, B. T., J. K. Walsh, K. Sexton, and S. A. Smitson. 1982. "Need Satisfaction in Narcolepsy." *Rehabilitation Literature* 43: 82-85.

Radloff, L. S., and B. T. Locke. 1986. "The Community Mental Health Assessment Survey and the CES-D Scale." In M. M. Weissman, J. K. Myers, and C. E. Ross, eds. *Community Surveys of Psychiatric Disorders*. New Jersey: Rutgers University Press, pp. 177-189.

Social Distance from Persons
with Narcolepsy
and Other Conditions

Felissa L. Cohen
Robyn W. Mudro

Both professional and nonprofessional groups generally tend to distance themselves from persons who are stigmatized for some reason (Albrecht, Walker and Levy 1982; Kalish 1966). Such reasons have included membership in stigmatized groups, including categories such as race, religion, contagious disease, mental illness, chronic illness and terminal illness. Stigma may result even from association (professional or other) with those in certain groups. This has been termed "courtesy stigma" by Goffman (1965). Social distance is most often described as the perceived degree of distance that one is comfortable placing between oneself and a designated person or group (Albrecht, Walker and Levy 1982; Bogardus 1933; Gentry 1986; Gentry 1987). The concept of social distance was first described in 1924 by Park, and the first reported investigation was by Bogardus in 1925 in his initial work on racial and ethnic minorities.

In 1933, Bogardus developed the Bogardus social distance scale in order to ascertain feelings about various ethnic groups. Since that time, various investigators have modified that scale. Gentry used a modification of it in her studies of homosexuality (Gentry 1986;

Felissa L. Cohen, RN, PhD, FAAN, is Director, Center for Narcolepsy Research, and Professor of Medical/Surgical Nursing, College of Nursing, University of Illinois at Chicago, Chicago, IL. Robyn W. Mudro, RN, MS, is Assistant Head Nurse, University of Illinois Hospital and Clinics, Chicago, IL.

This research was supported in part by Mr. J. A. Piscopo, founder and retired Chairman of the Board of Directors of Pansophic Systems, Inc.

Gentry 1987). In work on chronic illness, especially in HIV infection and AIDS, this scale was further modified (Cohen 1988).

Social distance is not an actual measure of spatial distances. Rather, it is related to the degree of understanding and intimacy that characterizes social relations (Park 1924). Tolerable social distance relates to the degree of comfort or discomfort experienced in a variety of situations. These reactions are distinguished from opinions (Gentry 1986). Such comfort or discomfort is related to social acceptance. For health professionals, the degree of perceived discomfort or perceived social acceptance of a person may influence direct patient care or the manner in which it is provided. The primary purpose of this study was to determine the social distance health professionals felt comfortable putting between themselves and persons with narcolepsy and other chronic conditions.

METHODS

The scale used in this study consisted of a continuum of six social distance conditions as developed by Cohen (1988) based on the work of Bogardus (1933) and Gentry (1986, 1987). These social distance categories represented degrees of closeness that characterized social relations and included city, neighborhood, church, casual acquaintance, close friend, and romantic interest on a continuum of increasing closeness. Validation of the distance intervals was done, and a pretest was conducted. Guttman scaling techniques were used. In order to meet the criteria for Guttman scaling, properties of unidimensionality and cumulativeness are required (SPSS 1983). A scale is considered to be unidimensional when all items measure distance from a single object such as the person with a specified chronic illness. Cumulativeness refers to scale items being ordered by degree of difficulty or on a continuum. A perfect Guttman scale is formed when all responses conform to a consistent pattern. In an ideal or perfect Guttman scale, a positive response to a closer-intimacy item such as acceptance of a person as a close friend would always be associated with positive responses to less intimate items such as admission of a person to the city in which the respondent lives. In order to determine if scale items conformed to these criteria, the appropriate statistics were performed. The coefficients of reproducibility and scalability, minimum marginal reproducibility and percent improvement exceeded minimum acceptable criteria for this type of scale (Cohen 1988; SPSS 1983).

The scale consisted of a continuum of categories with various degrees of social distance as described above. Participants were asked to check the social distance categories to which they would be comfortable in admitting persons with certain diseases or with specific characteristics.

For scoring, each item listed was assigned a score of 0 to 6, based on the number of categories checked for the specified condition. For example, a person who would be comfortable admitting a person with condition A only to their city receives a score of 1 while one who is comfortable in allowing all relationships including a romantic one receives a score of 6 for condition A. A lower score reflects a greater perceived degree of discomfort or lesser degree of comfort for that condition.

After obtaining the appropriate human subject consents, questionnaire packets consisting of the social distance scale discussed and demographic information were distributed randomly to nurses, pharmacists, laboratory technicians, and clergy at two large non-profit midwestern hospitals, one in a large urban center and one in a medium-sized city. All respondents were individually anonymous. Questionnaire packets were distributed in the fall of 1988 to 425 health professionals. Two hundred and nineteen were returned, for a response rate of 51.5%. This response rate exceeds the minimum needed for result confidence in this type of study (Babbie 1973).

RESULTS

The types of health professionals responding were mainly registered nurses. The majority of respondents were female. The mean age of respondents was 32.0 years (s.d. = 7.4) with the majority falling in the spread of 25 to 32 years of age. In regard to ethnic group, 83.1% were white, 3.2% black, 8.2% Asian and 2.7% Hispanic. Demographic characteristics of the respondents are shown in Table 1.

The means for the various conditions in the questionnaire, were analyzed. These are shown in Table 2, ordered from the closest or

TABLE 1

SOCIO-DEMOGRAPHIC CHARACTERISTICS OF SAMPLE

Variable	Frequency	Percent
Sex		
Male	46	21.0
Female	173	79.0
Marital status		
Never married	88	40.2
Married	105	47.9
Divorced	22	10.0
Separated	2	0.9
Widowed	1	0.5
Missing	1	0.5
Age Range		
17-24	22	10.0
25-32	106	48.4
33-40	52	23.7
41-48	17	7.8
49-57	11	5.0
Missing	11	5.0

TABLE 1 (continued)

Variable	Frequency	Percent
Ethnic Group		
White	182	83.1
Black	7	3.2
Hispanic	6	2.7
Asian	18	8.2
Other	2	0.9
Missing	4	1.8
Profession		
Registered Nurse	102	46.6
Pharmacist or Pharm. D.	35	16.0
Medical Lab Technologist	52	23.7
Clergy	28	12.8
Missing	2	0.9

least distant to the most distant. For narcolepsy the mean comfort level was just below the level of close friend. At the lowest end of the range was drug abuse, with respondents not quite allowing a drug abuser to live in their neighborhood.

It is interesting to note that the lowest mean scores were obtained for persons with conditions to which there might be a behavioral contribution or a degree of attribution of blame, for example, HIV

TABLE 2

SOCIAL DISTANCE MEANS FOR VARIOUS CONDITIONS*

CATEGORY	MEAN
Extra Digit on Hand	5.63
Diabetes Mellitus	5.63
Transplant Recipient	5.37
Epilepsy	5.33
Colostomy	5.31
Leukemia	5.27
Severe Acne	5.19
Hemophiliac	5.13
Dying of Incurable Illness	4.97
Narcolepsy	4.97
Chronic Pain	4.89
Depression	4.60
Genital Herpes	4.01
HIV Infected	3.80
Bisexual	3.76
Homosexual	3.75
AIDS	3.73
Promiscuous Person	3.54
Alcoholic	3.40
Ex-Convict	3.09
IV Drug Abuser	1.78

* Ordered from Least to Most Distant

infection, homosexuality, promiscuity, alcoholism, prison record, drug abuse.

Social distance means for narcolepsy were compared according to demographic variables. For most of these — sex, age as divided at/above the mean and below the mean, marital status, area of residence (large urban or medium-sized city), and professional group — there were no statistically significant differences noted in response to the person with narcolepsy.

In regard to length of time since graduation from their professional school, graduation time was divided at/above the mean and below the mean. Those who had graduated more recently (in the last eight years) from their professional education had higher mean social distance scores for narcolepsy, implying a closer perceived relationship than those who had graduated a longer time ago [$t(212) = 2.05$, $p = .04$]. Since there was no statistically significant relationship with age, these data suggest that perhaps in recent years, education of the health professional has included content and information allowing individuals to more effectively deal with their own feelings about persons with chronic illness.

The greatest difference in social distance perception of narcoleptics was seen in regard to the racial/ethnic group of respondents. The mean for white respondents for social distance scores for narcolepsy were 5.16 (s.d. = 1.08), while for all other racial groups it was 3.93 (s.d. = 1.69). A t test was again used for comparison. White respondents were more willing to allow a closer social distance than were nonwhite respondents. This difference was statistically significant [$t(213) = 5.43$, $p < .0001$]. Moreover, similar results were found for all the other chronic conditions that were not behaviorally associated in some way. Thus, in this study, health care professionals who were white would allow closer social distance between themselves and persons with chronic diseases and conditions that were *not* behaviorally related than would nonwhite health care professionals. Differences between the groups were not significant for those conditions and disorders that could be attributed to behavior such as promiscuity, HIV infection, AIDS, alcoholism, and drug abuse. Both white and nonwhite respondents maintained a similarly more distant social distance for those groups.

It could be argued that those persons who are nonwhite are more apt to be stigmatized than are whites. Thus, those who could themselves be seen as stigmatized did not allow a close social distance between themselves and persons with *any* of the chronic diseases or conditions listed that could bestow a "courtesy stigma."

When social distance means for persons with each of the chronic disease conditions were compared with that for narcolepsy, it was noted that persons with narcolepsy were the least accepted of the chronic illnesses, with the exception of genital herpes, depression, and HIV infection/AIDS, disorders which could be said to have some behavioral component. The reasons for this remain unclear.

CONCLUSIONS

This study found that health professionals would admit persons with narcolepsy to a social distance that was about equal to that of close friendship. However, this was among the most distant of the chronic illnesses listed. Nonwhite health professionals were more reluctant to permit a close relationship with persons having nonbehaviorally attributed conditions than were the white health professional respondents. Those respondents who had more recently completed their education were more comfortable with a closer perceived social distance to persons with narcolepsy than those who had graduated less recently. This suggests that continuing education programs dealing with the psychosocial components of narcolepsy and other chronic conditions might be useful in changing views in relation to desirability in social situations. If health professionals felt greater comfort toward persons with narcolepsy, this might carry over to more effective total care.

REFERENCES

Albrecht, G. L., V. G. Walker, and J. A. Levy. 1982. "Social Distance From the Stigmatized. A Test of Two Theories." *Social Science Medicine* 16:1319-1327.

Babbie, E. R. 1973. *Survey Research Methods*. Belmont, California: Wadsworth Publishing Co., Inc.

Bogardus, E. 1925. "Social Distance and Its Origins." *Journal of Applied Sociology* 9:216-226.

Bogardus, E. 1933. "A Social Distance Scale." *Sociology and Social Research* 17:265-271.

Cohen, F. 1988. "Perceived Social Distance From Persons With AIDS." Unpublished data.

Gentry, C. S. 1986. "Development of Scales Measuring Social Distance Toward Male and Female Homosexuals." *Journal of Homosexuality* 13:75-82.

Gentry, C. S. 1987. "Social Distance Regarding Male and Female Homosexuals." *Journal of Social Psychology* 127:199-208.

Goffman, E. 1965. *Stigma: Notes on the Management of Spoiled Identity.* Englewood Cliffs, New Jersey: Prentice-Hall.

Kalish, R. A. 1966. "Social Distance and the Dying." *Community Mental Health Journal* 2:152-155.

Park, R. E. 1924. "The Concept of Social Distance." *Journal of Applied Sociology* 8:339-344.

SPSS-X User's Guide. 1983. "Scalogram Analysis: Subprogram Guttman Scale." In *Statistical Package for the Social Sciences,* First edition. New York: McGraw-Hill Book Co., pp. 528-539.

Reported Accidents in Narcolepsy

Felissa L. Cohen
Carol E. Ferrans
Bruce Eshler

Accidents of any type cause distress to those involved. Accidents may result from no apparent cause or be precipitated by disease-related symptoms. Automobile accidents, in particular, exact a share of morbidity and mortality. In 1987, there were 47,297 deaths due to motor vehicle traffic accidents (National Center for Health Statistics 1990).

Excessive sleepiness while driving can result from insomnia, sleep apnea, shiftwork, narcolepsy, and many other disorders. In persons with narcolepsy, driving accidents have been described as resulting from excessive sleepiness, cataplexy, and visual disturbances. Persons with narcolepsy often report fighting drowsiness when driving.

Other investigators have reported upon driving in connection with narcolepsy and/or other disorders. Bartels and Kusakcioglu (1974) based their data on 105 narcoleptic respondents who drove and controls. Broughton and colleagues (1983) compared epileptics and narcoleptics with controls on a variety of parameters in relation

Felissa L. Cohen, RN, PhD, FAAN, is Director, Center for Narcolepsy Research, and Professor of Medical/Surgical Nursing, College of Nursing, University of Illinois at Chicago, Chicago, IL. Carol E. Ferrans, RN, PhD, is affiliated with the College of Nursing, University of Illinois at Chicago, Chicago, IL. Bruce Eshler is Research Specialist, Center for Narcolepsy Research, College of Nursing, University of Illinois at Chicago, Chicago, IL.

This research was supported in part by Mr. J. A. Piscopo, founder and retired Chairman of the Board of Directors of Pansophic Systems, Inc. The authors would like to thank the American Narcolepsy Association for its assistance with the data collection for this study.

to driving. The data from these studies are discussed later in this paper. Aldrich (1989) found in recent research that persons with sleep apnea and narcolepsy accounted for 71% of sleep-related accidents. Murray and Foley (1974) have reviewed the problem of the sleepy driver and the issues of prevention.

In this study, we examined the self-reported occurrence of automobile and other accidents in persons with narcolepsy and a control group from the general population.

METHODS

Subjects with narcolepsy were selected randomly from a mailing list obtained from the American Narcolepsy Association. This list included 13 states in the midsection of the United States. Of the 833 subjects to whom questionnaires were sent, 783 were eligible and locatable. A total of 3 mailings were done, and 539 returned the questionnaire, representing a 68.8% response rate. The control group from the general population was obtained through random selection from the Rockford, Illinois telephone directory. This city of 268,206 is considered an "all American city" and has been used in many research surveys. Of the 750 eligible and locatable persons to whom questionnaires were sent, 363 responded for a response rate of 48.4%.

RESULTS

Persons with narcolepsy were asked if they drive a car or not. Of the 530 responding to the question, 493 (93.0%) said that they did.

Reported Driving Accidents

Of those narcoleptics who stated that they drive a car, the number of driving accidents reported ranged from 0 to 22, with a mean of 1.87 (s.d. = 3.36). For those in the control group, the number of reported driving accidents ranged from 0 to 10 with a mean of 1.28 (s.d. = 1.48). The difference between the number of reported car accidents for those with narcolepsy and those in the general population was statistically significant [$t(725.3) = 3.43, p = .0006$].

Data comparing the number of driving accidents between those with narcolepsy and the controls are shown in Table 1.

For those narcoleptics who reported at least one accident, the mean number of accidents was 3.21 (s.d. = 3.89). The mean number of reported driving accidents for persons responding to the general population survey was 1.96 (s.d. = 1.41). This difference was statistically significant [$t(379.4) = 5.01$, $p = .0001$]. Thus, persons with narcolepsy reported more driving accidents than those persons in the comparison group.

Next, gender differences were examined for both the narcoleptics and the control group. The mean number of driving accidents reported by males and by females for both narcoleptics and controls were compared. The mean number of accidents for narcoleptic males was 2.35 (s.d. = 3.57), and for narcoleptic females the mean was 1.49 (s.d. = 3.16). This difference was statistically significant

TABLE 1. Driving Accidents Reported by Those with Narcolepsy and Controls[a]

No. Accidents	Narcoleptics (n=461)		Controls (n=323)	
	n	%	n	%
0	189	41.0	111	34.4
1	98	20.2	102	31.6
2	67	14.5	66	20.4
3	53	11.5	25	7.7
4	19	4.1	8	2.5
5	11	2.4	2	.6
more than 5	24	5.3	9	2.8

[a]Includes those currently driving only.

[t(489) = 2.83, p = .005]. Of the total sample, fewer females than males drove in both the control and narcoleptic groups.

Symptoms While Driving

Respondents were asked about symptoms experienced while driving and about both accidents and near accidents as a result of sleepiness while driving. First, narcoleptic persons will be compared to the control group. These data are summarized in Table 2. Of those responding, 74.8% of narcoleptics and 11.5% of the control group reported falling asleep while driving. This difference was statistically significant [$x^2(1) = 294.18, p < .0001$]. Respondents were then asked about experiencing sudden extreme weakness or cataplexy while driving. Only six persons in the control group reported such an experience, while among narcoleptics, 148 reported cataplexy while driving. Differences between these groups was again statistically significant [$x^2(1) = 100.85, p < .0001$].

Next, the narcoleptic respondents were examined in relation to gender. Of those narcoleptics who drove, 77.8% of the males and 67.9% of the females reported falling asleep while driving at some time. This difference between male and female drivers was statistically significant [$x^2(1) = 5.92, p = .015$]. Next, narcoleptic respondents were asked about experiencing sudden extreme weakness (cataplexy) while driving. Males reported slightly more cataplexy while driving than did females (32.6% vs. 26.8%), but the difference was not statistically significant (p > .05). This has been consistent with discussions of cataplexy found in the literature (Aldrich 1990; Guilleminault 1976) and our own data.

Symptoms and Driving Accidents

Actual and near driving accidents were investigated next. Driving accidents were compared between the control group and the narcoleptic respondents. These data are shown in Table 2. More narcoleptics reported actual car accidents due to sleepiness than did the control group respondents [21.1% vs. 2.2%]. This difference was statistically significant [$x^2(1) = 59.84, p < .004$].

Near car accidents due to sleepiness were examined. Far more narcoleptics as opposed to controls reported near driving accidents (55.6

TABLE 2. Reported Driving Effects in Narcoleptics and Controls in Percents

Reported Effect	Narcoleptics	Controls
Fell asleep	74.8	11.5[a]
Weakness/Cataplexy	30.0	1.9[b]
Near accidents	55.6	11.1[c]
Accidents	21.1	2.2[d]

[a] p < .0001

[b] p < .0001

[c] p < .0001

[d] p = .004

75

vs. 11.1%). This difference was statistically significant $[x^2(1) = 158.44, p < .0001]$.

Consequences of Driving Accidents

Driving accidents have potential consequences other than physical injury. When the narcoleptic and control groups were compared, 7.9% of narcoleptics and 2.5% of the general population reported higher insurance rates due to driving accidents, and this difference was statistically significant $[x^2(1) = 8.27, p = .004]$. Only two of the males with narcolepsy, and none of the females, reported ever having had their driver's license suspended due to driving accidents. When the narcoleptic and control groups were compared, there were no statistically significant differences between the two groups (two narcoleptics and five respondents from the general population).

Comparisons

The results of this study in relation to driving effects and narcolepsy, compared with the results of Bartels and Kusakcioglu (1965) and Broughton and colleagues (1983) are shown in Table 3.

Other Accidents

Respondents were asked whether sleepiness or other symptoms of narcolepsy had led to other types of accidents besides automobile accidents, either at home or at work. About one-third (165 respondents) indicated that this had occurred. Next, they were asked to describe the type of accident that had occurred. Of those specifically designated, the most frequently occurring were falls followed by burns from objects other than cigarettes, cuts, breaking things, cigarette burns, and spills. These data are shown in Table 4. For most of these reported accidents, there were no statistically significant differences between male and female respondents except for burns from hot pots and objects. Not surprisingly, significantly more females than males reported this accident $[x^2(1) = 9.16, p = .002]$.

TABLE 3. Comparison of Driving Effects on Narcoleptics in Percents

	Cohen	Bartels[a]	Broughton[b]
Fell asleep	74.8	77.0	72.7
Weakness	30.0	-	34.1
Near accident	55.6	-	63.6
Accidents	21.1	16.0	34.1
Higher rate of insurance	7.9	-	15.9
Suspended licence	0.4	-	5.0

[a] Bartels, E. C. and O. Kusakcioglu. 1965. "Narcolepsy: A Possible Cause of Automobile Accidents." *Lahey Clinic Foundation Bulletin* 14:22-26.

[b] Broughton, R., Q. Ghanem, Y. Hishikawa, Y. Sugita, S. Nevsimalova, and B. Roth. 1983. "Life Effects of Narcolepsy: Relationships to Geographic Origin (North American, Asian or European) and to Other Patient and Illness Variables." *The Canadian Journal of Neurological Sciences* 10:100-104.

TABLE 4. Accidents Described by Narcoleptics[a,b] (n = 165)

ACCIDENTS	No.	%
Falls	61	36.9
Burns from hot pots and objects other than cigarettes	24	14.5
Cuts from knife, saw, etc	21	12.7
Breaking things	17	10.3
Burns from cigarettes	8	4.9
Spilling things	8	4.9
Fell asleep while smoking	4	2.4

Accidents of poor judgment	3	1.8
Poured food out into nothing	3	1.8
Others[c]	77	46.7

Near drowning
Sewed through finger
Electrical shocks
Minor accidents
Choked on food
Wrecked factory machine
Shaving cuts
Burned child
Burned clothing
Frostbite

[a]Driving accidents excluded
[b]Those describing at least one accident
[c]Selected examples listed

CONCLUSIONS

Accidents, both with automobiles and others, continue to plague persons with narcolepsy to a greater degree than controls. Reported actual and near driving accidents occurred significantly more frequently in persons with narcolepsy than in the control group. Nearly 75% of persons in this study reported that they had fallen asleep while driving as compared to 11.5% of controls. Thirty percent of persons with narcolepsy had experienced cataplexy while driving. The most commonly reported household accident was falls, which were experienced by nearly 37% of persons with narcolepsy who reported accidents.

NOTE: This study did not differentiate between accidents that were reported before and after diagnosis of narcolepsy or between those that occurred before or after effective treatment. Data are being presently analyzed from another survey conducted by the first author to address these issues.

REFERENCES

Aldrich, M. S. 1990. "Narcolepsy." *The New England Journal of Medicine* 323(6):389-394.

Aldrich, M. S. 1989. "Automobile Accidents in Patients With Sleep Disorders." *Sleep* 12(6):487-494.

Bartels, E. C, and O. Kusakcioglu. 1965. "Narcolepsy: A Possible Cause of Automobile Accidents." *Lahey Clinic Foundation Bulletin* 14:22-26.

Broughton R., Q. Ghanem, Y. Hishikawa, Y. Sugita, S. Nevsimalova, and B. Roth. 1983. "Life Effects of Narcolepsy: Relationships to Geographic Origin (North American, Asian or European) and to Other Patient and Illness Variables." *The Canadian Journal of Neurological Sciences* 10:100-104.

Guilleminault, C. 1976. "Cataplexy." In C. Guilleminault, W. C. Dement, and P. Passouant, eds. *Narcolepsy: Advances in Sleep Research*. New York, NY: Spectrum, pp. 125-143.

Murray, T. J. and A. Foley. 1974. "Narcolepsy." *Canadian Medical Association Journal* 110:63-66.

National Center for Health Statistics. 1990. *Vital Statistics of the United States*. 1987, vol. II, part A. Washington: Public Health Service.

Sexual Dysfunction in Men with Narcolepsy

Ismet Karacan
Nilgun Gokcebay
Max Hirshkowitz
Mine Ozmen
Ercan Ozmen
Robert L. Williams

Men with narcolepsy syndrome frequently experience erectile problems. Sexual incapacity devastates some patients psychologically and renders them impotent in nonsexual endeavors as well (Cohen 1988; Kales et al. 1982; Karacan 1982; Roth 1980). Notwithstanding the undeniable psychosocial importance of human sexuality, it has received limited recognition in comparison to other aspects of health. In men, sexual dysfunction most often involves erectile failure.

Cultural indoctrination, psychosocial factors, and interpersonal

Ismet Karacan, MD, DSc (Med), ACP, is Director, Sleep Disorders and Research Center, Department of Psychiatry, Baylor College of Medicine, Houston, TX. Nilgun Gokcebay is affiliated with the Sleep Disorders and Research Center, Department of Psychiatry, Baylor College of Medicine, and Sleep Research Laboratory, Research Service, Veterans Affairs Medical Center, Houston, TX. Max Hirshkowitz, PhD, is Associate Clinical Director, Sleep Disorders and Research Center, Department of Psychiatry, Baylor College of Medicine, and Associate Director, Sleep Research Center, Veterans Affairs Medical Center, Houston, TX. Mine Ozmen is affiliated with the Sleep Disorders and Research Center, Department of Psychiatry, Baylor College of Medicine, and Sleep Research Laboratory, Research Service, Veterans Affairs Medical Center, Houston, TX. Ercan Ozmen is affiliated with the Sleep Disorders and Research Center, Department of Psychiatry, Baylor College of Medicine, and Sleep Research Laboratory, Research Service, Veterans Affairs Medical Center, Houston, TX. Robert L. Williams is affiliated with the Sleep Disorders and Research Center, Department of Psychiatry, Baylor College of Medicine, and Sleep Research Laboratory, Research Service, Veterans Affairs Medical Center, Houston, TX.

dynamics between the patient and his mate can each play a role in producing or exacerbating erectile failure. Many cultures, including our own, attribute great importance to sexual prowess, either overtly, as part of peer group pressure, or in more subtle ways. The role attributed to males by the society puts additional pressure on the sexually incapable man and this can provoke severe deterioration of self image, depression, or both. The psychosocial effects of erectile failure often depend on a complex interaction of several variables. These include personality factors, harmony or disharmony in the couple's relationship, coexisting medical or psychiatric illnesses, and the severity of the problem.

The reported prevalence of sexual dysfunction in patients with narcolepsy varies greatly, ranging from 17% (Roth 1980) to 67% (Guilleminault, Carskadon, and Dement 1974). Broughton and Ghanem (1976) found 39% of patients with narcolepsy complained of impotence. Most were being treated with antidepressant and stimulant medications. A remarkably similar prevalence estimate (38%) was reported by Takahashi (1976) in a group of patients with narcolepsy syndrome who were treated with tricyclic antidepressants. Roth (1980) also mentioned that Vein found sexual problems in 20% of cases. Sampling biases taken into consideration, one might conservatively estimate the prevalence of sexual dysfunction in narcoleptics at approximately 25%.

The origins of narcolepsy-related impotence may vary. Among possible etiologies are (1) erectile dysfunction secondary to sleepiness, (2) concomitant diabetes mellitus, (3) sexual arousal-induced cataplexy, and (4) pharmacotherapeutically-induced iatrogenic impotence. More theoretically, under-release of dopamine in the brainstem may represent the biological substrate for impotence in narcolepsy syndrome.

LOSS OF LIBIDO SECONDARY TO SLEEPINESS

Severe sleepiness can result in loss of sexual and libidinal drive. Excessive daytime sleepiness is the cardinal symptom of narcolepsy. Some investigators conceptualize impotence among patients with sleep apnea as secondary to hypersomnolence, depression, or both (Hudgel 1986). A similar pattern may be present in men with narcolepsy syndrome. Acute sleep deprivation produces hypersexuality, whereas chronic sleep loss is more often correlated with loss of sexual interest and depression. The following case illustrates the relationship between sleepiness and sexual dysfunction.

Case History — CMH

> Mr. H., a 73-year-old, retired gentleman, had trouble with excessive daytime sleepiness since the age of 15 years. He could not resist sleepiness during sedentary activity or during exciting situations. This included sexual activity. He displayed a classic picture of narcolepsy, with short and refreshing daytime naps, hypnagogic hallucinations, and infrequent cataplectic episodes induced by laughter. Evaluation at our sleep disorders and research center confirmed the diagnosis of narcolepsy with very short sleep latencies and sleep-onset REM episodes on both nights and during multiple sleep latency tests. A treatment trial was arranged that included the use of methylphenidate and protriptyline. Excessive daytime sleepiness has been a life-long problem for this patient that has impaired his social life, libido, and consequently his sexual functioning.

Nervous system changes are associated with sleepiness and can be documented with pupillometry. Dark-adapted, normally alert individuals maintain fairly stable pupillary diameter when observed for 10 minutes. Typically, the pupil's diameter is seven or more millimeters. Sleep-deprived subjects, insomnia patients, and individuals with narcolepsy have large pupillary oscillations (Schmidt and Fortin 1982). Erectile function, mediated by the autonomic nervous system, can likewise be compromised by changes in sympathetic-parasympathetic balance associated with sleepiness.

DIABETES MELLITUS

Perhaps the most intriguing developments in research concerning the etiology of narcolepsy was the recent connection found between this disease and the HLA DR2 antigens. Initial investigation of human leukocyte antigens was prompted in part by the observation of a greater incidence of non-insulin dependent diabetes (NIDD) among patients with narcolepsy syndrome than in the normal population (Honda et al. 1986). The relationship between diabetes and erectile failure is well established and presumably results from a combination of neurogenic and vascular dysfunctions. Abnormalities among impotent men with diabetes include impaired autonomic nervous system function, prolonged sacral spinal reflex latencies, penile vascular insufficiency, and reduced nocturnal penile tumescence (Karacan and Hirshkowitz 1988). An increased incidence of NIDD among men with narcolepsy consequently produces a greater probability of organic impotence among these patients. The following case is characteristic of the association between narcolepsy syndrome and diabetes mellitus.

Case History — EJK

> Mr. K., a 55-year-old, retired gentleman, presented with the complaint of erectile failure that had developed after years of normal functioning. Mr. K. was diagnosed with narcolepsy 20 years ago and with diabetes mellitus 14 years ago. His erectile dysfunction began approximately 10 years ago. Initially he attributed his erectile difficulties to methylphenidate which was prescribed for his sleepiness, and he discontinued the medication seven years ago. However, after discontinuing his medication, daytime sleepiness worsened and there was no change in his sexual function. Our evaluation at the sleep disorders and research center revealed short sleep latencies during nocturnal polysomnography and sleep-onset REM episodes on all naps. His nocturnal penile erections were clearly impaired. At the time of evaluation the patient was taking insulin. After evaluation he was advised to resume methylphenidate therapy.

SEXUAL AROUSAL-INDUCED CATAPLEXY

Cataplexy, the sudden loss of tone in certain muscle groups, exists in 60-65% of patients with narcolepsy. Cataplexy, when present in narcolepsy, is usually provoked by intense emotions. These may include anger, arousal, and joy. This feature of narcolepsy syndrome may initially seem unrelated to sexual function; however, in some patients it poses a serious problem. In our clinical practice, we have encountered several cases in which sexual arousal, as an intense emotional stimulus, induced cataplectic episodes. The following patient vignette illustrates this circumstance.

Case History-PW

> Mr. W., a 33-year-old man, had a 14-year history of excessive daytime somnolence. His sleepiness caused serious social and professional problems in his life, including discharge from the United States Army, multiple revocation of his driver's license, and loss of several jobs. He was unemployed at the time of evaluation. Aside from severe sleepiness, he experienced sudden loss of muscle tone upon sexual arousal. This greatly disrupted relationships with his sexual partners, resulting in his inability to attain a stable intimate relationship. These attacks of cataplexy also occurred during other exciting situations (e.g., laughing and running). Mr. W. experienced unpleasant visual and tactile hallucinations while falling asleep. He had previously seen several physicians for the problem and had attempted different treatments, without success. Our evaluation revealed two sleep-onset REM periods during multiple sleep latency testing and short sleep latencies on both nights. He was diagnosed as having narcolepsy and a combination of methylphenidate and imipramine (for cataplexy) was recommended.

PHARMACOTHERAPEUTICALLY-INDUCED ERECTILE DYSFUNCTION

Iatrogenic impotence is common in men with narcolepsy. The medications currently used to treat narcolepsy can be classified as either central nervous system stimulants prescribed to relieve daytime sleepiness and tricyclic antidepressants administered to reduce cataplexy.

Dextroamphetamine, pemoline, methylphenidate, and mazindol are the stimulants usually prescribed to maintain alertness during the daytime. Little is known regarding the relationship between their chronic use and erectile function; in addition, the existing research has produced controversial results. There is, however, evidence that chronic use of other central nervous system stimulants, amphetamine in particular, interferes with sexual function and provokes erectile failure, ejaculatory problems, and altered libido (Segraves et al. 1985; Wheatley 1983). These deteriorations in sexual physiology presumably result from the parasympatholytic and anticholinergic properties of the drug.

Case History — PO

> Mr. O., a 59-year-old businessman, had trouble remaining awake while driving and eating. He also had a propensity for falling asleep during the daytime. His complaints dated back 30 years. Frequent short naps produced refreshment. He also reported "weak spells" during exciting situations, and vivid imagery and muscular weakness at sleep onset. He was diagnosed as narcoleptic and administered methylphenidate seven years ago. Five years ago he began experiencing difficulty obtaining and maintaining penile erection. He related his erectile problem to the medication. Our evaluation substantiated the diagnosis of narcolepsy; sleep-onset REM was found on both nights and during all naps. Polysomnograms indicated his sleep-related erections were impaired. We recommended alternation between methylphenidate and scheduled short periodic naps, with napping preferred to stimulant use, when possible.

The notoriously adverse effects of tricyclic antidepressant medications on erectile function are fairly well appreciated (Segraves et al. 1985). Even though the exact mechanism by which these drugs adversely affect erectile function is still a matter of debate, it is widely accepted that the anticholinergic effects are responsible for impotence. This parasympathetic blockade varies between the different tricyclic compounds.

Case History — MW

> Mr. W., a 32-year-old, married man, had a history of excessive daytime sleepiness for the past 10 years. He also reported sudden weakness in certain muscle groups when he became extremely excited. Two years after the onset of his complaints, he was diagnosed as having narcolepsy and dextroam-

phetamine was prescribed. This medication provided relief, initially. However, it became ineffective after several months. His complaints were severe enough to require hospitalization and gradual withdrawal from dextroamphetamine. While hospitalized, a regimen of methylphenidate and imipramine was established. Subsequently, he began to experience problems obtaining erection and a decrease in his sexual desire. The patient related the onset of his sexual problems to the medications he was taking. We evaluated the patient polysomnographically, both while he was taking the medications and six days after he discontinued them. Recordings indicated improved nocturnal penile tumescence after cessation of drug therapy. We advised alternation between medication use and scheduled naps and modification of lifestyle to accommodate more daytime naps.

The clinician should never underestimate the importance of a treatment's adverse effect on sexual function. Erectile impotence has major effects on patients' marital and social life. The willingness to accept this side effect and the ability to adapt to the change varies greatly between individuals and couples. Practitioners should be aware of the possibility of noncompliance with agents interfering with erectile function, as has been associated with antihypertensive therapy (Hogan, Wallin and Baer 1980). Indeed Gillin, Horowitz and Wyatt (1976) noted that some patients with narcolepsy may have discontinued their medication because it interfered with sexual activity.

DOPAMINE THEORY

One of the more widely accepted theories of the etiology of narcolepsy is that it results from widespread under-secretion of dopamine in the central nervous system with hypersensitivity to acetylcholine (Mitler, Nelson and Hajdukovic 1987). It is well known that patients with Parkinson's disease, who suffer from lack of dopamine in basal ganglia, frequently have sexual dysfunction. A number of investigations implicate dopamine in the mediation of sexual behavior. Studies indicate that apomorphine (in rats), bromocryptine (in hyperprolactinemic men), and L-DOPA (in men with Parkinson's disease) can enhance sexual function or partially alleviate erectile dysfunction (Segraves et al. 1985; Wheatley 1983). Moreover, clinical trials are currently underway assessing the therapeutic efficacy of an investigational central dopamine agonist for the treatment of sexual dysfunction in men and women. It is not yet resolved whether dopamine-related changes in sexual function are direct central nervous system effects, indirect consequences of changes in hormonal regulation, or some combination of these and other effects. Nonetheless, as a corollary to the dopamine under-release theory, one could postulate that the pathophysiology underlying narcolepsy contributes directly to erectile impairment.

SUMMARY AND CONCLUSIONS

Men with narcolepsy syndrome frequently experience erectile problems. The exact prevalence is difficult to assess given sampling biases in groups studied; however, 25% may serve as a conservative estimate. We know from our experience in the sexual dysfunction clinic that the psychosocial effect of sexual incapacity can range from complete acceptance to severe deterioration of self-image. Cultural indoctrination concerning male potency, personality factors, and interpersonal dynamics between the patient and his mate all play a role.

We reviewed possible etiologies of impotence in men with narcolepsy syndrome. Central dopaminergic effects, loss of libido secondary to sleepiness, concomitant diabetes mellitus, cataplexy induced by sexual arousal, and pharmacotherapeutically induced iatrogenic impotence were discussed. We presented several case vignettes to help illustrate some of these factors.

Included in the consensus report of the International Symposium on Narcolepsy held in 1985 was a mandate for further research concerning sexual dysfunction associated with narcolepsy; however, little work has been done. For instance, since in clinical practice patients are usually dispensed antidepressants, stimulants, or both, iatrogenic effects on sexual function are partially unavoidable. Therefore, the timing of attempted sexual activity may be crucial. We suspect, as in the example of cardiovascular medication (Ware 1984), blood drug levels are lower, and penile erections are less impaired toward morning before the next dose is taken. At this time, in addition to being refreshed, the patient should be less affected by the anticholinergic properties of the tricyclic compound, and consequently be able to obtain better quality erections. It is our clinical impression that this strategy is beneficial for some patients; however, no formal clinical trial has been conducted to validate this notion. Similarly, the tricyclic antidepressants with fewer anticholinergic side-effects are presumed to interfere less with erectile function; however, systematic data are needed. Given the number of patients afflicted and the social, marital and psychological consequences of sexual dysfunction on a patient's life, we believe that the sexual problems associated with narcolepsy syndrome demand more attention.

REFERENCES

Broughton, R. and Q. Ghanem. 1976. "The Impact of Compound Narcolepsy on the Life of the Patient." In C. Guilleminault, W. C. Dement, and P. Passouant, eds. *Narcolepsy*. New York: Spectrum, pp. 201-220.

Cohen, F. L. 1988. "Narcolepsy: A Review of a Common, Life-Long Disorder." *Journal of Advances in Nursing* 13:546-556.

"Consensus Statement from the Second International Symposium on Narcolepsy." 1986. *Sleep* 9:290-291.

Gillin, J. C., D. Horowitz, R. J. Wyatt. 1976. "Pharmacologic Studies of Narcolepsy Involving Serotonin, Acetylcholine, and Monoamine Oxidase." In C. Guilleminault, W. C. Dement, and P. Passouant, eds. *Narcolepsy*. New York: Spectrum, pp. 585-604.

Guilleminault, C., M. Carskadon, and W. C. Dement. 1974. "On the Treatment of Rapid Eye Movement Narcolepsy." *Archives of Neurology* 30:90-93.

Hogan, M. J., J. D. Wallin, and R. M. Baer. 1980. "Antihypertensive Therapy and Male Sexual Dysfunction." *Psychosomatics* 21:234-237.

Honda, Y., Y. Doi, R. Ninomiya, C. Ninomiya. 1986. "Increased Frequency of Non-Insulin Dependent Diabetes Mellitus Among Narcoleptic Patients." *Sleep* 9:254-259.

Hudgel, D. 1986. "Clinical Manifestations of the Sleep Apnea Syndrome." In E. C. Fletcher, ed. *Abnormalities of Respiration During Sleep*. New York: Grune and Stratton, pp. 21-37.

Kales, A., C. R. Soldatos, E. O. Bixler, A. Caldwell, R. J. Cardieux, J. M. Verrechio, and J. D. Kales. 1982. "Narcolepsy-Cataplexy." *Archives of Neurology* 39:169-171.

Karacan, I. 1982. "Managing Marital Conflicts Associated with Sleep Disorders." *Medical Aspects of Human Sexuality* 16:71-94.

Karacan, I. and M. Hirshkowitz. 1988. "Erectile Dysfunction Associated with Diabetes." In S. Smirne, M. Franceschi, and L. Ferini-Strambi, eds. "Sleep in Medical and Neuropsychiatric Disorders." Milano: Masson.

Mitler, M. M., S. Nelson, and R. Hajdukovic. 1987. "Narcolepsy: Diagnosis, Treatment, and Management." *Psychiatric Clinics of North America* 10:593-606.

Roth, B. 1980. *Narcolepsy and Hypersomnia*. Basel: S. Karger.

Schmidt, H. S. and L. D. Fortin. 1982. "Electronic Pupillography in Disorders of Arousal." In C. Guilleminault, ed. *Sleeping and Waking Disorders: Indications and Techniques*. Menlo Park, CA: Addison-Wesley, pp. 127-143.

Segraves, R. T., R. Madsen, C. S. Carter, and J. M. Davis. 1985. "Erectile Dysfunction Associated with Pharmacological Agents." In R. T. Segraves and H. W. Schoenberg, eds. *Diagnosis and Treatment of Erectile Disturbances: A Guide for Clinicians*. New York: Plenum, pp. 23-63.

Takahashi, S. 1976. "The Action of Tricyclics (Alone or in Combination with Methylphenidate) upon Several Symptoms of Narcolepsy." In C. Guilleminault, W. C. Dement, and P. Passouant, eds. *Narcolepsy*. New York: Spectrum, pp. 625-641.

Ware, J. C. 1984. "Suppression of NPT During the First REM Sleep Period." *Sleep Research* 13:71.

Wheatley, D. 1983. *Psychopharmacology and Sexual Disorders*. New York: Oxford University Press.

Psychosocial Aspects of Narcolepsy in Children and Adolescents

Neil B. Kavey

The psychosocial aspects of narcolepsy in children have not received much attention because it is unusual for narcolepsy to be diagnosed in childhood. Yoss and Daly (1960) reported that out of 400 patients seen at the Mayo Clinic with the diagnosis of narcolepsy, only 4% were 15 years of age or younger. At the Stanford sleep disorders center, Guilleminault (1987) reported that, over a ten-year period, they were referred only five patients between ages 7 and 11 with *suspected* narcolepsy. The center at Henry Ford Hospital in Detroit (Young et al. 1988) reported on eight narcoleptics age 15 or younger, two of whom were under 12 years of age, and there are three isolated case reports in the literature (Wittig et al. 1983; Carskadon, Harvey, and Dement 1981; Chisholm et al. 1985). However, this is not to say that narcolepsy rarely occurs in children. The insidious onset of sleepiness obscures the actual time of onset of the disorder so that we do not actually know the incidence of diagnosable narcolepsy in childhood. In the Yoss and Daly sample (1960), in which only 4% of the narcoleptics were age 15 or younger, 26% of narcoleptics reported having symptoms by age 10, about 40% had symptoms before the onset of puberty (estimated age 12) and 59% had symptoms by age 15. Navelet, Anders, and Guilleminault (1976) reported that excessive sleepiness was recognized in 20% of their patients before age 11, and 49% had symptoms by age 16. Even in adolescence, which is the most common time for the disorder to begin, diagnosis goes unestablished for years.

Neil B. Kavey, MD, is Director, Sleep Disorders Center, Columbia-Presbyterian Medical Center and Associate Clinical Professor of Psychiatry, College of Physicians and Surgeons, New York, NY.

Daytime sleepiness in childhood and adolescence is far more commonly due to sleep apnea or inadequate hours of sleep than to narcolepsy. In sleep apnea and insufficient sleep, the age of onset of daytime sleepiness may be much earlier than in the youngest narcoleptics. Children with either apnea or insufficient sleep can have sleepiness even in the first year of life. Few narcoleptics describe sleepiness before age six.

The classic symptoms of narcolepsy are not different in childhood than in adulthood. They include sleepiness, cataplexy, hypnagogic hallucinations and sleep paralysis, and they occur with the same incidence in children and adults. Disturbed nocturnal sleep is also common in both age groups, possibly even more so in the pediatric group (Young et al. 1988). Possibly there is a difference in the timing of the onset of the symptoms. While excessive daytime sleepiness is usually the first symptom reported in children and adults, Young et al. (1988) reported that the associated symptoms seemed to begin in closer association with the onset of excessive daytime sleepiness in children than in adults.

While any of the associated symptoms could be terrible for children to experience, probably the most devastating symptoms for psychosocial development are sleepiness and cataplexy, with sleepiness usually being the more devastating. By multiple sleep latency (MSLT) examination (Young et al. 1988), narcoleptic children had a higher mean total number of REM onsets and a shorter average sleep latency than their adult counterparts. This means that children may be even sleepier than their adult counterparts, a point that highlights the importance of early diagnosis. But with the subtlety of the onset of the disorder, early diagnosis could be exceptionally difficult. Young children might fail to recognize in themselves the abnormality of the sleepiness they feel and fight off, living through years of their lives with a subtle cloud of sleepiness that they find uncomfortable but assume is normal because they have nothing with which to compare it. Adolescents will manufacture explanations for the way they feel, often disparaging themselves, and adults will far more often be critical of the child's or adolescent's behavior than concerned about its possibly being a symptom. Their sleepiness could even appear to be just a normal variant until it becomes extreme, especially in adolescents, who are so often sleepy due to unmet sleep needs. By the time the narcolepsy is recognized, the toll among children and adolescents could be enormous.

An awareness of the consequences of daytime sleepiness on the psychosocial development of children must be and rarely is considered when making treatment decisions for children with apnea. (Usually the decision to do a tonsillectomy and adenoidectomy or not is based on the severity of the apnea or straining.) The degree of sleep fragmentation and the question of whether the child is showing signs of daytime sleepiness are not considered of primary importance compared to the cardiac issues. Yet the psychiatric consequences could be severe.

While never getting the attention that diagnostic and treatment issues get, the psychosocial aspects of narcolepsy have not been completely ignored. Broughton and his colleagues published reports in the early 1980s of questionnaire surveys comparing narcoleptics of different cultures (1981, 1983) and comparing narcoleptics with epileptics (1984). Rogers (1984) gathered data from a series of interviews. Both documented marked effects on work, education, driving, recreation, and social functioning. Broughton concluded that the symptom most strongly affecting the narcoleptics' lives was the daytime sleepiness. A few reports discussed the incidence of psychiatric symptoms (Kales et al. 1982; Wilcox 1985; Krishnan et al. 1984; Rogers 1984).

This paper will discuss psychosocial problems that could be encountered by young narcoleptics. Some of the material will apply to children with sleep apnea as well and should be considered in the decision of whether or not to aggressively treat an apneic child.

The first task is to list those areas in which one would expect problems. Just being aware of potential problems equips professionals to better deal with them, to teach coping strategies, to deal with the inevitable problems and frustrations, and to make sound decisions about treatment.

I have chosen to focus on problems that could arise due to the sleepiness and cataplexy caused by the disorder itself. I am not discussing how treatment might modify those problems, what problems result from the treatment or its limitations, or what difficulties result from a child or adolescent having to endure the problems of having *any* serious illness or disorder.

The problems I am going to emphasize are not problems for all or probably even most narcoleptics. What problems narcoleptics face and how well they are equipped to deal with them depends to a good extent on when the disorder started to affect alertness. An important question is when, in the life cycle, subtle manifestations of the disorder started to take effect. The earlier in life the symptom, the more devastating the effects. Some of the difficulties narcoleptics have coping with their symptoms occur because the sleepiness of early years compromised the development of mature coping systems and a healthy sense of self and others. The impact of even the best parenting and schooling is limited when integrated or distorted by a mind affected by sleepiness. The ideas presented here are derived from interviews with narcoleptics and their families, including extensive interviews with a nine year old's mother and a twelve year old and her mother.

SOCIAL PROBLEMS IN CHILDHOOD

Problems Related to Sense of Self and Others

1. In the sleepy state, children are less responsive to others than they are when fully alert.
2. Others are less responsive to children in the sleepy state than to alert children. The whole manner in which children relate to children and adults could be affected. Adults, especially, will relate more positively to a smiling, alert, and responsive child than to a child dulled by sleepiness. Parents might fail to understand their own child and could be angry and frustrated with the child's seeming apathy. Exchanges between parents and child might be fraught with misinterpretations. The entire way one perceives oneself and relates to people and one's environment is affected by the level of alertness. The quality of that crucial resonance between people is affected. Facial expressions, intonations, events, the physical environment, are all subject to interpretation. The child's, preadolescent's, and adolescent's view of the world could all be formed by a brain dulled by sleepiness.
3. One's perception of oneself, one's self-image and one's

sense of oneself as being likeable, liked, or popular can be negatively affected. How good one feels about oneself and how popular one is depend very much on the nature of those crucial interactions with others. When relationships suffer, so does self-esteem.

4. Narcoleptics are vulnerable to feeling different from others. In some ways the sleepy child *is* different. For example, a sleepy child does not feel the same way about an experience as does an alert child and might wonder why people seem to get so much pleasure out of something that looks quite mundane through sleepy eyes. A narcoleptic with cataplexy may actually try to avoid feelings in order to avoid cataplexy. Hypnagogic hallucinations and sleep paralysis can be terrifying to a child and can leave him or her feeling "crazy" and strange.

5. A child who is different is likely to be picked on. But being victimized might just as much be due to an awkward social manner, for reasons mentioned above, as to the presence of symptoms. Nevertheless, daytime sleepiness is hard to hide, and the child who falls asleep on the school bus, in assemblies, and in class is going to be subject to ridicule. And self-defense in such situations may be difficult; just accepting the challenge of a fight could end in the embarrassment of collapsing to the floor in a cataleptic attack.

Problems with Social Functioning

6. The narcoleptic might show an inability to function in social settings others enjoy, such as going to movies, reinforcing the feeling of being different.

7. Both coordination and athletic performance could be compromised. A sleepy child might regularly or periodically have his or her performance affected by the lack of alertness. Baseball can be a difficult game for someone who is falling asleep in the field or in the dugout. Cataplexy could have devastating effects on sports performance. Collapse during exciting moments could lead to frustration and discouragement. Exciting

moments in tennis, track or sport could end in defeat caused by a cataplectic attack.

8. The disorder will certainly affect the activities in which the child chooses to be involved. He or she is sure to choose those that can be done with the least chance of failure and embarrassment.

Problems with Mood and Family

9. Children could both look and be depressed as a result of the above problems. Psychiatric help over and above basic support and guidance may be necessary. Although making an early diagnosis is crucial in avoiding problems and teaching coping strategies, one may or may not be successful in altering the symptoms, and establishing the diagnosis does not necessarily result in an alleviation of all problems.

10. Parent-child interaction will be affected. Parents' difficulty dealing with a child's sleepiness and seeming apathy before the disorder is diagnosed has already been mentioned. After the diagnosis is established, parents will experience disappointment, guilt, and concern. They may find it difficult to let a child develop any independence because of his or her vulnerability to accidents or abuse.

11. Parents of other children could even inadvertently contribute to the narcoleptic's feeling of being different. Understanding nothing about narcolepsy and cataplexy, other children's parents might be reluctant to include the narcoleptic child in social activities for fear the child will have an "attack."

12. The diagnosis is obviously going to influence parents' and teachers' selections of activities for the child. Restrictions will inevitably result, at times in ways quite visible to peers. No one is going to let a child with cataplexy climb the ropes in gym.

Problems at School

13. Learning difficulties are likely (Aguirre, Broughton, and Stuss 1985). It is hard to learn, memorize and retain information gathered through a haze of sleepiness, and it is easy to miss

not only presented facts but crucial integrative statements that are so important if students are to understand the overall theme of what is being taught that day.

14. Narcoleptic students may appear to teachers to be disinterested and careless. Students may miss such important information as an announcement of an assignment or a test.

15. Feeling sleepy and falling asleep in tests can occur. In later grades, tests get longer and the possibility of falling asleep increases.

16. Failing, or at least relative failure, can result when efforts to study lead not to achievement but to sleepiness and confusion. In the earlier years, compromised scores in tests of intelligence and basic skills can influence parents' and teachers' overall evaluation of a child's abilities. Fifty-one percent of Broughton's (1981) adult patients remembered sleepiness causing poor grades in school. Affected children must often deal with the feeling that they are stupid or lazy, feelings that destroy self-esteem and could affect interest in pursuing advanced schooling. They could be mislabeled as learning disabled and in many ways could test out similarly.

17. Children with narcolepsy could be labeled as behavior problems. To overcome sleepiness, a child could become disruptive. Sleepy children can even appear hyperactive. Self-consciousness about the condition could also cause a child to show off and be disruptive.

18. Probably the most serious consequence, although the most avoidable, could be teachers' anger and frustration at the child's sleepiness. It can be difficult for a teacher to feel positively about a student who sleeps in class. Prior to diagnosis, a child's sleepiness is likely to antagonize teachers. Fifty-one percent of Broughton's (1981) patients felt they had interpersonal problems with teachers because of their symptoms. Even after diagnosis is made, however, a teacher is likely to feel that the student could stay awake in class if he or she were really interested. It is easier to understand a student falling asleep in another teacher's class than in one's own.

SOCIAL PROBLEMS IN ADOLESCENCE

The psychological and social problems of developing or having narcolepsy or any form of excessive daytime sleepiness in adolescence are in some ways different from the problems one would expect for younger children. As mentioned above, the earlier one develops sleepiness, the more likely one is to develop core psychological problems. On the other hand, adolescence has its own set of special conditions, and some problems are unique to adolescence. Adolescence is the most common time for narcolepsy to begin to manifest itself. All of the problems mentioned above could and do occur in adolescence. Below are additional problems specific to this age.

1. The lack of resonance between a sleepy teenager and his or her friends brings with it a set of problems quite different from earlier years. The teenage years are special years for identifying with people outside the home and for forming friendships that help one move out of the home. Sleepiness can make this stage of development almost impossible.

2. Social awkwardness could be a problem. It could be very difficult to feel on top of, or involved in, social situations when one is falling asleep at parties or dances or, again, on the school bus. Falling asleep on a date or during some sexual activity might seem humorous to others, but for those who have been horrendously embarrassed by their sleepiness for years, that would be no laughing matter. The nodding adolescent with drooping eyes may be seen as weird or even as a drug abuser. In fact, the narcoleptic adolescent may find stimulating drugs make him or her feel more normal, and thus could become a drug abuser.

3. Interest, involvement, and performance in activities and athletics could be affected, as could enthusiasm for activities that others are involved in. It could be difficult for a narcoleptic to stay awake in school club meetings, and performance in athletic events or other visible activity is likely to be highly variable and therefore avoided. Working after

school to earn extra money could present the problem of getting to the job safely as well as holding the job.

4. Affected adolescents may experience dejection, depression, or the need to overcompensate.

5. Parents of a sleepy teenager are likely to be overprotective and may not be willing to let their child engage in activities in which being sleepy could be dangerous. In their desire to protect, they could frustrate healthy attempts to separate.

6. The problems with driving are evident. There are risks even for a fully alert teenager, and the dangers are very much greater for a sleepy one. Not only is there the added risk of a sleepy person driving, but also the parents' extra anxiety and resulting restrictions.

7. Although teenagers are not allowed to drink, that does not always stop them, and drinking can increase sleepiness, resulting in even more awkward and dangerous situations.

8. Problems with sexuality could easily result, as an insecure and sleepy adolescent is more likely to make injudicious sexual decisions than a fully alert teen.

9. Learning problems and difficulty in concentrating, experienced by affected children at earlier ages, are likely to be even greater at this age because of the increased demands placed on the older student. Books are longer and reading material more difficult. Students must concentrate for longer periods, and tests are longer. The college board examinations, for example, are hours long.

10. Unless a student is particularly gifted, it is almost inevitable that test scores are not going to be what they could be. In high school, career aspirations and choices are going to be affected by this.

11. Because of all the above, narcoleptics are likely to have limited chances for college and academic success.

12. Increased self-image problems are almost inevitable, considering the pressures put on adolescents to perform. They face such problems as feeling that they cannot keep up with the demands of upper grades. Parents and teachers tell them how disappointed they are with their poor marks.

It should be understood that the above problems are all ones to which childhood narcoleptics are vulnerable. Depending on individual good fortune, a young person could escape with few of the mentioned difficulties. Early diagnosis is probably the best means of insuring that children troubled with excessive daytime sleepiness learn sound coping mechanisms and avoid the spiraling problems that sleepiness can cause in the young.

REFERENCES

Aguirre, A., R. Broughton, and D. Stuss. 1985. "Does Memory Impairment Exist in Narcolepsy-Cataplexy?" *Journal of Clinical and Experimental Neuropsychology* 7(1):14-24.

Broughton, R., Q. Ghanem, Y. Hishikawa, Y. Sugita, S. Nevsimalova, and B. Roth. 1981. "Life Effects of Narcolepsy in 130 Patients from North America, Asia and Europe Compared to Matched Controls." *Canadian Journal of Neurological Science* 8(4):299-304.

Broughton, R., Q. Ghanem, Y. Hishikawa, Y. Sugita, S. Nevsimalova, and B. Roth. 1983. "Life Effects of Narcolepsy: Relationships to Geographic Origin (North American, Asian or European) and to Other Patient and Illness Variables." *Canadian Journal of Neurological Science* 10:100-104.

Broughton, R. J., A. Guberman, and J. Roberts. 1984. "Comparison of the Psychosocial Effects of Epilepsy and Narcolepsy/Cataplexy: A Controlled Study." *Epilepsia* 25(4):423-433.

Carskadon, M. A., K. Harvey, and W. C. Dement. 1981. "Multiple Sleep Latency Tests During the Development of Narcolepsy." *Western Journal of Medicine* 135:414-418.

Chisholm, R. C., C. J. Brook, G. F. Harrison et al. 1985. "Prepubescent Narcolepsy in a Six-Year-Old Child." *Sleep Research* 15:113.

Guilleminault, C. 1987. "Narcolepsy and Its Differential Diagnosis." In C. Guilleminault, ed. *Sleep and Its Disorders in Children*. New York: Raven Press, pp. 181-194.

Kales, A., C. R. Soldatos, E. O. Bixler, A. Caldwell, R. J. Caieux, J. M. Verrechio, and J. D. Kales. 1982. "Narcolepsy-Cataplexy II: Psychosocial Consequences and Associated Psychopathology." *Archives of Neurology* 39:169-171.

Krishnan, R. R., M. R. Volow, P. P. Miller, and S. T. Carwile. 1984. "Narcolepsy: Preliminary Study of Psychiatric and Psychosocial Aspects." *American Journal of Psychiatry* 141(3):428-431.

Navelet, Y., T. Anders, and C. Guilleminault. 1976. "Narcolepsy in Children." In C. Guilleminault, W. C. Dement, and P. Passouant, eds. *Narcolepsy*. New York: Spectrum, pp. 171-177.

Rogers, A. E. 1984. "Problems and Coping Strategies Identified by Narcoleptic Patients." *Journal of Neurosurgical Nursing* 16(6):326-334.

Wilcox, J. 1985. "Psychopathology and Narcolepsy." *Neuropsychobiology* 14:170-172.

Wittig, R., F. Zorick, T. Roehrs, J. Sicklestell, and T. Roth. 1983. "Narcolepsy in a Seven-Year-Old Child." *Journal of Pediatrics* 102:725-727.

Yoss, R. E. and D. D. Daly. 1960. "Narcolepsy in Children." *Pediatrics* June: 1025-1033.

Young, D., F. Zorick, R. Wittig, T. Roehrs, and T. Roth. 1988. "Narcolepsy in a Pediatric Population.' *AJDC* 142:210-213.

ADDITIONAL READING

Carskadon, M. A., E. J. Orav, and W. C. Dement. 1983. "Evolution of Sleep and Daytime Sleepiness in Adolescents." In C. Guilleminault and E. Lugarese, eds. *Sleep/Wake Disorders: Natural History, Epidemiology, and Long-Term Evolution*. New York: Raven Press, pp. 201-216.

SECTION II:
LEARNING AND COGNITIVE DEVELOPMENT IN PERSONS WITH NARCOLEPSY

Can We Predict Cognitive Impairments in Persons with Narcolepsy?

Karen M. Smith
Sharon L. Merritt
Felissa L. Cohen

The evidence for self-perceived cognitive impairment in narcoleptic persons is consistent and compelling. Broughton et al. (1981) found that 48.9% of narcoleptic respondents reported their memory

Karen M. Smith, PhD, is Senior Research Specialist, Center for Narcolepsy Research, College of Nursing, University of Illinois at Chicago, Chicago, IL. Sharon L. Merritt, RN, EdD, is Assistant Director, Center for Narcolepsy Research, College of Nursing, University of Illinois at Chicago, Chicago, IL. Felissa L. Cohen, RN, PhD, FAAN, is Director, Center for Narcolepsy Research and Professor of Medical/Surgical Nursing, College of Nursing, University of Illinois at Chicago, Chicago, IL.

This research was funded in part by Mr. J. A. Piscopo, founder and retired Chairman of the Board of Directors of Pansophic Systems, Inc. The American Narcolepsy Association assisted in the data collection for Study 2.

had worsened since development of narcolepsy. Of these, 81.0% reported deterioration of their memory for recent events, and 10.1% reported poor memory for remote events. Of those who were employed, job difficulties were ascribed to memory problems by 31.2% and to poor concentration by 42.6%. Among matched controls, only 9.4% reported memory problems, and job difficulties were attributed to poor memory or poor concentration by 9.3% and 11% respectively. Similar findings were described by Broughton and Ghanem (1976), and Broughton, Guberman and Roberts (1984). Memory and concentration problems have also been cited by narcoleptic interviewees as major causes of decreased educational performance (Rogers 1984).

Laboratory tests of memory and cognitive function among narcoleptic subjects, however, have not produced such clear results. When tested in the laboratory using standard measures of both short- and long-term memory, narcoleptic patients have not been shown to have any significant memory impairment (Aguirre, Broughton and Stuss 1985; Broughton 1982; Broughton et al. 1986; Valley and Broughton 1981). Consistently, the only demonstrable performance deficit found in persons with narcolepsy has been with prolonged, monotonous tasks requiring sustained attention (Billiard 1976; Broughton 1982; Broughton et al. 1986; Godbout and Montplaisir 1986; Guilleminault and Dement 1977; Mitler, Gujavarty, Sampson and Browmar 1982; Rogers 1986; Valley and Broughton 1981, 1983), a finding that has been ascribed to chronic drowsiness (Broughton et al. 1986) or to repeated microsleep episodes (Guilleminault and Dement 1977). To date there have been no studies which examined memory deterioration over a span longer than 20 minutes, nor have there been attempts to differentiate among learning, retention, and retrieval processes (Spear 1978). In the first study described here, these memory functions were assessed and a battery of neuropsychological tests was used to evaluate a number of cognitive functions that might be impaired by narcolepsy.

In the second study, self-reports of learning and memory problems from a large survey of narcoleptic respondents were correlated with specific symptom reports and personal characteristics, indicating that some symptom profiles in narcolepsy are more likely to be associated with experienced cognitive deficits than are others.

STUDY 1:
LEARNING AND MEMORY
IN NARCOLEPTIC SUBJECTS AND CONTROLS

Twenty-four narcoleptic patients, median age 57, and 24 control subjects, matched for age, sex, and education, were each tested twice in the laboratory. Half of each group returned for Session II one day after Session I, the other half returned after one week. Narcoleptic subjects were asked to continue their normal medication and sleep routine, and when possible were scheduled at the time of day that they normally felt most alert.

All subjects filled out a background questionnaire, including 19 items on symptom severity, rated on a five-point scale. They also answered questions on medications and health history, and on lateral preferences for use of one hand, foot and eye.

A word list learning and memory procedure consisting of five free recall learning trials, recall after 25 minutes, recall after the delay, followed by a recognition trial, and five relearning trials was completed by all subjects. In addition, a battery of neuropsychological tests was administered. These tests were chosen to reflect the functions of verbal processing, verbal fluency, cognitive flexibility, word retrieval, mental tracking, response planning, and response inhibition. Tests included the Halstead-Reitan Trailmaking Test (Lezak 1983; Weintraub and Mesulam 1985), parts A and B; the Go-No Go Test (Weintraub and Mesulam 1985); the Boston Naming Test (Kaplan, Goodglass and Weintraub 1983); the Revised Token Test, subtests IV, VIII, IX and X (McNeil and Prescott 1983) the Mental Tracking-Alphabet (subjects recited the alphabet backwards starting with the letter R); Mazes 7, 8, and 9 from the Wechsler Intelligence Scale for Children (WISC) (Lezak 1983); the Controlled Oral Word Association Test (Lezak 1983); the Stroop Color Word Test (Golden 1978); and Mental Tracking-Subtraction (subjects subtracted from 100 by sevens for ten subtractions).

Subjects also rated their subjective sleepiness on a Visual Analog Sleepiness (VAS) Scale three times in each session.

RESULTS

In the initial 5 learning trials, controls made significantly more correct responses, and in the second session the narcoleptic subjects showed a significantly greater gap between recognition and recall (Cohen and Smith 1989). There were no significant differences in adjusted recall scores for Session II, in number of words recognized, in number or type of recognition errors, in number of recall errors, or in the relearning curves, nor were there Group by Delay interactions. Learning behavior during the initial five trials also differed, with controls making more responses of all types during these trials, repeating words already recalled more often, and having a smaller proportion of responses that were correct, unrepeated recalls of the words on the list (Cohen and Smith 1989).

On the neuropsychological testing, there were no significant differences found between groups. Within the narcoleptic group, however, there were significant correlations between severity scores on symptom scales and performance scores on a number of tests. In particular, severity of ocular symptoms (double vision, blurred vision, and drooping eyelids) and muscular symptoms ("restless legs" at night and muscle spasms) were significantly related to tests of mental function as summarized in Table 1.

When the narcoleptic group was divided into Low and High Ocular Symptom severity groups using a median split at a score of 5, a number of interesting contrasts emerged. The High Ocular Symptoms group had significantly poorer scores ($p < .05$, by t-test) on mean number correct during word list learning and relearning, had worse word retrieval scores, and had a lower response rate than did the Low Ocular Symptoms group. They had lower fluency scores on the Controlled Oral Word Association Test, made more errors on the Revised Token Test, took more time on all cards of the Stroop Test, made more errors in Mental Tracking Alphabet, and took more time to complete Mental Tracking-Subtraction. An exception to the general picture of poor performance among High Ocular Symptoms subjects was in number of errors made on WISC Maze

Table 1. Symptom Severity and Performance: Narcoleptic Group

Symptom Scale	Task	r^*
Ocular Symptoms Scale		
	Mental Tracking-Alphabet	
	(errors)	.594
	Stroop Word Card	.673
	Stroop Color Card	.550
	Stroop Color-Word Card	.585
	Stroop Interference Score	.544
	Word Association-letter F	-.601
	Word Association-total fluency	-.542
	VAS Sleepiness Scale #2	-.603
	VAS Sleepiness Scale #3	-.525
Muscular Symptoms Scale		
	Mental Tracking-Alphabet	
	(time to completion)	.699
	(number of pauses)	.621
	Stroop Word Card	.535
	VAS Sleepiness Scale #4	-.559

* All r's significantly different from 0, $p < .01$, two-tailed.

9, on which this group did significantly better. This task had the greatest demands for spatial processing of any in our battery, along with minimal verbal demands. In contrast, the tasks on which the High EYE group did worse were those with strong components of verbal fluency and verbal and sequential processing.

The Low and High EYE severity groups did not differ significantly on age, education, or sex distribution, but the High EYE group did report higher mean severity scores for current depression $(3.69 \pm .86$ vs. $2.45 \pm .93, t (22) = 3.39, p = .003$), and excessive daytime sleepiness $(3.85 \pm .99$ vs. $2.54 \pm .82, t (22) = 3.47, p = .002$).

Educational level was significantly correlated with performance of a number of tasks for both groups, especially the Boston Naming Test, both Mental Tracking tasks, fluency in Word Association, the Stroop Test, and errors on the Revised Token Test (r's from .52 to .81, $p < .01$). For the control group, only Trailmaking scores were significantly correlated with educational level. With the exception of one learning trial in the narcoleptic group, none of the word list learning and memory scores were correlated with educational level for either group. Age was not correlated with any performance scores for the narcoleptic group. In the control group, a significant relationship between age and performance was found on one score derived from the Controlled Oral Word Association Test ($r = .59, p < .01$).

Within the narcoleptic group, only two performance scores were associated with any measure of subjective sleepiness, and only one of these, time taken to read the Stroop Test word card, was correlated with a VAS rating taken in the same session ($r = -.53, p < .01$). No statistical association was found between EDS ratings and any performance score.

STUDY 2:
NARCOLEPSY INFORMATION
QUESTIONNAIRE (NIQ)

The NIQ was a mail survey of 700 respondents from the nationwide patient registry of the American Narcolepsy Association. A complete description of the sample and methods for this questionnaire will be found in "Learning Style Preferences of Persons with Narcolepsy," elsewhere in this volume.

The symptom items from the NIQ were grouped into a number of symptom scales, as before. Those of interest here are:

1. Learning and Memory (LRNMEM): difficulty learning and concentrating, memory problems and forgetfulness;
2. Visual Disturbances (VIS): blurred vision, double vision, difficulty focusing, eye flickering, eye fatigue, drooping eyelids, seeing haloes around objects, sensitivity to certain kinds of light;
3. Daytime sleepiness (DAYSLEEP): sleep attacks and excessive daytime sleepiness.

Also included in analyses of self-reported cognitive impairment were item scores on nocturnal disturbance, cataplexy, sleep paralysis, hypnagogic hallucinations and muscle spasms. A summary depression score, CES-D (Radloff 1977), was also employed, along with data on age, sex, and education.

Self-reported problems with learning and memory were common in this sample, as in previous studies. Moderate or severe problems with memory were reported by 38.6%; with forgetfulness by 39.6%, with concentration by 40.4%, and with learning by 26.27%.

Men and women did not differ on overall LRNMEM scores, but women did rate their memory problem as more severe (1.4 ± 1.04 vs. 1.2 ± 1.01, t (675) = 2.19, p = .029). Level of educational achievement was not significantly correlated with any of these scores. Age, however, did have a strong relationship to self-reported cognitive problems, showing a significant declining linear trend with increasing age.

LRNMEM was also significantly intercorrelated with a number of other symptom ratings, as well as with CES-D depression scores. Multivariate methods were used to identify the most powerful predictors of this measure of cognitive impairment. A hierarchical multiple linear regression was performed using LRNMEM as the dependent variable, with independent variables entered in stepwise fashion. To be retained in the solution, a variable had to be entered with an F value with $p = .05$ or less, and also had to account by itself for a significant ($p < .05$) portion of the residual variance at that step.

The significant predictors for LRNMEM were found to be VIS, CES-D, and DAYSLEEP, which together accounted for 31.45% of the variance in LRNMEM.

DISCUSSION

The evidence from Study 1 suggests that narcoleptic persons may learn, consolidate, and store information as well as controls, but they may be less able to retrieve that information from long-term memory stores. Anecdotal reports of the memory problems of persons with narcolepsy do often follow the theme of being unable to dredge up from memory some fact that the person "should know very well." Knowing that the "memory" problems in narcolepsy may in fact be retrieval problems could prove useful in characterizing brain dysfunction in narcolepsy.

Although cognitive impairment may be experienced as global, the actual functional effects can be very limited in scope. The neuropsychological tests chosen for Study 1 surveyed several narrow areas of mental function, specifically those requiring verbal processing, verbal fluency, cognitive flexibility, word retrieval, mental tracking, response planning, and response inhibition. None of these produced any statistically reliable differences between narcoleptic subjects and matched controls, although the self-rated difficulties in memory and concentration were much greater in the narcoleptic group.

Within the narcoleptic group, there was a clear association between severity of ocular and muscular symptoms and poorer performance on tasks requiring verbal fluency, and verbal and sequential processing. Ocular symptoms, in turn, were closely related to self-rated depression and excessive daytime sleepiness. Since most tests in this study made strong verbal processing demands, we cannot say to what extent the problems associated with ocular symptoms restricted the verbal aspect of these tests. One intriguing finding was the superior performance of those with severe ocular symptoms on Maze 9, a task with great demands for accurate spatial processing.

A greater range of tasks, with greater representation of nonverbal function, might give a clearer idea of how ocular symptoms might be related to the cognitive impairment in narcolepsy.

Multivariate analysis of self-ratings in Study 2 provided converging evidence that a cluster of symptoms, notably ocular problems, depression and, to a certain extent, daytime sleepiness may distinguish those narcoleptics with cognitive problems from those without. Despite the existence of a clear age trend in self-reported learning and memory problems in Study 2, age did not enter the regression equation developed here. This implies that any age effect is indirect, resulting from declining age trends found in other predictors, especially ocular symptoms and depression. The question of whether narcoleptic persons with severe depression, ocular symptoms, or muscular symptoms also have greater physiological sleep tendency would be well worth following up.

There was some evidence that persons with narcolepsy may utilize compensatory strategies or functions to deal with cognitive difficulties. In word list learning in Study 1, our narcoleptic subjects had a high rate of response efficiency, more often pinpointing correct, unrepeated words from the list than did the controls. Despite their lower scores during learning trials, narcoleptic subjects obtained recall scores not significantly different from those of the controls, indicating that the material may have been learned equivalently by both groups. Also, within the narcoleptic group, those who reported severe ocular symptoms seemed to have a disadvantage on tasks requiring verbal fluency and verbal and sequential processing, but performed better on a task requiring a high level of spatial processing. On this task — Maze 9 — the narcoleptics with severe ocular problems also performed significantly faster than their matched controls (2.64 ± 1.0 min vs. 4.59 ± 2.9 min, paired t $(11) = 2.76, p = .018$).

In Study 2, narcoleptic respondents had attained a fairly high level of educational achievement, with over half (55.6%) having attended college. Of those working 30 or more hours per week, 64.4% were employed in technical, professional, or managerial occupations, jobs that usually require certain competence in thinking, learning and memory.

CONCLUSIONS

Can we predict cognitive impairment among persons with narcolepsy? The answer must be qualified by the limited range of cognitive functions measured so far in our research program, but some generalizations can be made. First, it seems that the narcoleptic persons most likely to suffer cognitive impairment will be those who experience depression and/or severe ocular symptoms. These people are more likely to be young, since depression and ocular symptoms are both reported to be more severe in younger narcoleptic persons.

What specific impairments will these persons experience? Persons with narcolepsy as a group may experience difficulties retrieving material from memory, although so far this has only been demonstrated for recently-learned verbal material. Persons with severe ocular symptoms seem to have trouble with tasks requiring verbal fluency and verbal and sequential processing. The possibility of compensatory learning strategies and cognitive functions among persons with narcolepsy may be worth pursuing.

REFERENCES

Aguirre, M., R, Broughton, and D. Stuss. 1985. "Does Memory Impairment Exist in Narcolepsy-Cataplexy?" *Journal of Clinical and Experimental Neuropsychology* 7:14-24.
Billiard, M. 1976. "Competition Between the Two Types of Sleep, and the Recuperative Function of REM Sleep versus NREM Sleep in Narcoleptics." In C. Guilleminault, W.C. Dement, and P. Passouant, eds. *Narcolepsy: Advances in Sleep Research*. New York: Spectrum, pp. 77-96.
Broughton, R. 1982. "Performance and Evoked Potential Measures of Various States of Daytime Sleepiness. *Sleep* 5(Suppl):S135-S146.
Broughton, R. and Q. Ghanem. 1976. "The Impact of Compound Narcolepsy on the Life of the Patient." In C. Guilleminault, W.C. Dement, and P. Passouant, eds. *Narcolepsy: Advances in Sleep Research*. New York: Spectrum, pp. 201-219.
Broughton, R., Q. Ghanem, Y. Hishikawa, Y. Sugita, S. Nevsimalova, and B. Roth. 1981. "Life Effects of Narcolepsy in 180 Patients from North America, Asia and Europe Compared to Matched Controls." *Canadian Journal of Neurological Sciences* 8:299-304.
Broughton, R.J., A. Guberman, and J. Roberts. 1984. "Comparison of the Psy-

chosocial Effects of Epilepsy and Narcolepsy/Cataplexy: A Controlled Study." *Epilepsia* 25:423-433.

Broughton, R., V. Valley, M. Aguirre, J. Roberts, W. Suwalski, and W. Dunham. 1986. "Excessive Daytime Sleepiness and the Pathophysiology of Narcolepsy-Cataplexy: A Laboratory Perspective." *Sleep* 9:205-215.

Cohen, F. L. and K.M. Smith. 1989. "Learning and Memory in Narcoleptic Patients and Controls." *Sleep Research* 18:117.

Godbout, R. and J. Montplaisir. 1986. "All-Day Performance Variations in Normal and Narcoleptic Subjects." *Sleep* 9:200-204.

Golden, C.J. 1978. *Stroop color and word test*. Chicago: Stoelting Co.

Guilleminault, C. and W.C. Dement. 1977. "Amnesia and Disorders of Excessive Sleepiness." In R.R. Drucker-Colin and J.L. McGaugh, eds. *Neurobiology of Sleep and Dreaming*. New York: Academic Press, pp. 439-456.

Kaplan, E., H. Goodglass, and S. Weintraub. 1983. *Boston Naming Test*. Philadelphia: Lea and Febiger.

Lezak, M.D. 1983. *Neuropsychological Assessment*. New York: Oxford University Press.

McNeil, M.R. and T.E. Prescott. 1983. *Revised Token Test*. Austin: Pro-Ed.

Mitler, M.M., K.S. Gujavarty, M.G. Sampson, and C.P. Browman. 1982. "Multiple Daytime Nap Approaches to Evaluating the Sleepy Patient." *Sleep* 5(Suppl.):S119-S127.

Radloff, L.S. 1977. "The CES-D Scale: A Self-Report Depression Scale for Research in the General Population." *Applied Psychological Measurement* 1:385-401.

Rogers, A.E. 1984. "Problems and Coping Strategies Identified by Narcoleptic Patients." *Journal of Neurosurgical Nursing* 16: 326-334.

Rogers, A. 1986. "Memory Deterioration versus Attentional Deficits in Patients with Narcolepsy." *Sleep Research* 15:418.

Spear, N.E. 1978. *The Processing of Memories: Forgetting and Retention*. Hillsdale, NJ: Lawrence Erlbaum, Associates.

Valley, V. and R. Broughton. 1981. "Daytime Performance Deficits and Physiological Vigilance in Untreated Patients with Narcolepsy-Cataplexy Compared to Controls." *Revue d' Electroencephalographie et de Neurophysiologie Clinique* (Paris) 11:133-139.

Valley, V. and R. Broughton. 1983 "The Physiological (EEG) Nature of Drowsiness and its Relation to Performance Deficits in Narcolepsy." *Electroencephalography and Clinical Neurophysiology* 55:243.251.

Weintraub, S. and M-M. Mesulam. 1985. "Mental State Assessment of Young and Elderly Adults in Behavioral Neurology." In M-M. Mesulam, ed. *Principles of Behavioral Neurology*. Philadelphia: F.A. Davis Company, pp. 71-123.

Learning Style Preferences
of Persons with Narcolepsy

Sharon L. Merritt
Felissa L. Cohen
Karen M. Smith

People with narcolepsy often complain of significant learning and memory problems that, presumably, are related to excessive daytime sleepiness and sleep attacks (Broughton and Ghanem 1976; Cohen 1988; Kales et al. 1982; Rogers 1984). Decreases in alertness level affect the ability of people with narcolepsy to attend to learning tasks. For example, during a sleep attack, people may concentrate on trying to stay awake rather than on the learning at hand. However, when investigators compared the cognitive abilities of narcoleptics to those of matched controls, little evidence was found in laboratory settings to confirm differences in memory abilities (Aguirre, Broughton and Stuss 1985; Roberts and Rosenberg 1990). People with narcolepsy report using a variety of strategies in academic settings to adapt their learning behaviors to daytime sleeping difficulties (Rogers 1984).

Learning style has been defined as the ways that people prefer to behave in a learning situation (Merritt 1989). In contrast with cog-

Sharon L. Merritt, RN, EdD, is Assistant Director, Center for Narcolepsy Research, College of Nursing, University of Illinois at Chicago, Chicago, IL. Felissa L. Cohen, RN, PhD, FAAN, is Director, Center for Narcolepsy Research, and Professor of Medical/Surgical Nursing, College of Nursing, University of Illinois at Chicago, Chicago, IL. Karen M. Smith, PhD, is Senior Research Specialist, Center for Narcolepsy Research, College of Nursing, University of Illinois at Chicago, Chicago, IL.

This research was funded in part by Mr. J. A. Piscopo, founder and retired Chairman of the Board of Directors of Pansophic Systems, Inc. The authors wish to thank the American Narcolepsy Association for its assistance in carrying out this research.

115

nitive ability, learning style assessment is concerned with assessing people's preferences for the various ways of learning that can be present in a teaching-learning situation. Learning style theorists postulate that people are more motivated to learn and learn better when taught according to their learning style preferences (Messick 1984). People with narcolepsy may be required to select particular ways of learning in order to cope with their reported memory and concentration difficulties. This study was designed to determine if people with narcolepsy differed in their preferences for learning in patient education situations as defined by the Canfield learning style model (Canfield 1980, 1988), and if these differences were related to personal characteristics, symptom experiences and right/left motor skills, and cognitive thinking patterns. Little is known about the learning patterns of narcoleptics. This information could provide data to health care professionals for designing patient education instruction that is more congruent with the coping abilities people with narcolepsy use in learning situations.

CANFIELD MODEL OF LEARNING STYLE

The Canfield Model of Learning Style (1980, 1988) is concerned with describing individual differences in preferences for selected conditions and some sensory modes commonly found in learning situations. The four conditions and four modes which influence learning responsiveness are outlined in Figure 1. Canfield developed the Learning Style Inventory (LSI), which consists of eight scales based on these conditions and modes. Scores for each scale are obtained by summing the RANKS assigned to the 12 items associated with each condition and the six items associated with each mode. The LSI was designed to be used with a young adult college student population and therefore is not suited specifically to measuring learning preferences associated with patient education situations. Additionally, the ranking method used to score the instrument means that the instrument is an ipsative one, since scores assigned items are dependent upon their relationship (rank) with respect to other items (Merritt and Marshall 1984).

Patient Learning Style Questionnaire (PLSQ), based on the Canfield model, was constructed by one of the authors. The PLSQ con-

FIGURE 1. Canfield's Model of Learning Style

Affiliation	Friendly relations with <u>peers</u> and <u>instructor</u>
Structure	<u>Organized</u> instruction with <u>detailed</u> information about learning requirements
Achievement	Setting <u>own</u> <u>goals</u> and learning <u>independently</u>
Eminence	Authoritative, <u>expert</u> instructor who <u>controls</u> learning situation
Listening	<u>Verbal</u> instruction
Reading	<u>Print</u> media
Iconics	<u>Visual</u> presentation
Direct Experience	<u>Experiments</u> and learning <u>exercises</u>

tains items placed within the context of patient education and uses a normative Likert scale rating format for measuring preferences for four conditions and four modes of learning.

METHODS

Design and Sample

This retrospective, descriptive study was conducted with a convenience sample of 700 respondents with narcolepsy out of 1140 patients who were chosen randomly from the registry of the American Narcolepsy Association (ANA) (61.4% response rate). A five-part questionnaire, the Narcolepsy Information Questionnaire (NIQ), was prepared for mailing by Center for Narcolepsy staff and shipped to ANA, where staff addressed and mailed the NIQ. The names of people with narcolepsy who were asked to participate were unknown to the investigators. A reminder postcard (two weeks after initial mailing) and a second questionnaire (one month later) were sent to nonrespondents. Participation was deemed non-risk by the University's Institutional Review Board, since materials were returned voluntarily and anonymously.

Instrumentation

The Narcolepsy Information Questionnaire (NIQ), a 5-part self-administering instrument, was designed to collect the following information from the narcoleptic respondents (Figure 2):

1. *Part I—Background data*—personal demographic characteristics and experience with a comprehensive list of symptoms developed from research literature that describes the health complaints of people with narcolepsy;
2. *Part II—Right/Left motor patterns*—a handedness score obtained with the Briggs-Nebes Handedness Inventory (Briggs and Nebes 1975), and an overall laterality score that was derived from the average for the handedness items plus ratings for a foot and an eye preference;
3. *Part III—Patient Learning Styles Inventory* (PLSQ)—eight learning style scale scores (four conditions and four modes)

obtained by summing Likert-type ratings assigned items associated with the various scales (1 = important for learning to 4 = unimportant for learning) (Merritt, in press);

4. *Part IV — Right/Left thinking patterns* — a right/left hemisphere thinking pattern score obtained with the ALERT scale of thinking (Crane, no date);

5. *Part V — Center for Epidemiologic Studies — Depression* (CES-D) — a depressive symptomatology score obtained from the sum of ratings assigned 20 items that were derived from a review of general purpose and depression psychiatric inventories.

Scores for the PLSQ are the dependent variables in this report. Information from other portions of the NIQ were used as independent measures, i.e., as grouping variables or variables examined for their influences on learning style scale scores.

Characteristics of the Sample

The majority of narcoleptic respondents were between 41 and 55 years of age, female, white, married, lived in a suburban/rural geographic region, worked at least part-time, had 30 or more years of work experience, and were employed at the professional/technical/ managerial occupational level (Table 1). In terms of educational experiences, the majority had at least a high school diploma or its equivalent, had completed formal schooling at least 20 years earlier, had participated in some type of learning classes since graduation but five years or more had elapsed since their participation, and had learned about narcolepsy by reading about this disorder on their own (Table 2).

Analysis of variance and Scheffe posthoc test results revealed that there were significant differences in the preferences of people with narcolepsy for various conditions and modes of learning (Figure 3). The respondents prefer *structured* learning that includes detailed information about what is to be learned. Organized instruction that provides detail concerning the learning requirements may help people with narcolepsy compensate for their attention and memory difficulties.

Although significantly lower than the structure preference, the

FIGURE 2. Narcolepsy Information Questionnaire (NIQ)—Independent Measures

NIQ Section I

Personal Background (5 items) - age, sex, education, occupation, income

Narcolepsy Symptom Categories - sum of ratings (0-3) for items associated with each category as follows:

Classic (4 items) - excessive daytime sleepiness (EDS), cataplexy, sleep paralysis, hypnagagic hallucinations

New Classic (1 item) - classic score plus nighttime sleeping difficulties

Associated (3 items) - automatic behavior, snoring, nightmares

Other (3 items) - sleepwalking, muscle spasms, visual disturbances

Learning/Memory (4 items) - difficulties concentrating and learning, forgetfulness, memory problems

NIQ Section II. R/L Motor Patterns

Handedness (12 items) [a] - sum of ratings assigned each item from - 2 (left) to + 2 (right)

Laterality (average of 12 items plus 2 items) - average handedness score plus foot and eye preferences

NIQ Section III. ALERT Thinking Scale (20 item) [b] - sum of 20 two option items scored 1 for left and 2 for right.

NIQ Section IV. Center for Epidemiologic Studies - Depression (CES-D) Scale (20 items) - sum of ratings assigned each item from 0-3.

[a] Source: Briggs & Nebes, 1975.
[b] Source: Loren Crane, Western Michigan State University, no date.

Table 1. Personal Demographic Characteristics

Variable	N	%	Variable	N	%
Age			**Work Status**		
18-40	108	16.82	Not working	345	49.71
41-55	215	33.49	1-29 hrs./wk	83	11.96
56-65	185	28.82	30 hrs. or more	266	38.33
66 & older	129	20.09			
			Years of Work		
Sex			**Experience**		
Male	261	38.44	Less than 1 yr.	15	2.19
Female	418	61.56	1-9 yrs.	114	16.64
			10-19 yrs.	145	21.17
Ethnicity			20-29 yrs.	134	19.56
American Indian	10	1.50	30 yrs. or more	277	40.44
Black	27	4.06			
White	617	92.78	**Occupational Level**		
Oriental	3	.45	Prof/Tech/Manage	361	52.86
Spanish American	8	1.20	Cler/Sales/Service	174	25.48
			Farm/Fish/Forest	8	1.17
Marital Status			Process/Mach/Bench/		
Single	92	13.49	Structure	51	7.47
Married	428	62.76	Other	89	13.03
Widowed	50	7.33			
Separated	9	1.32	**Number People Support**		
Divorced	103	15.10	Self only	350	55.91
			2	172	27.48
Geographic Area			3	49	7.83
Inner City	91	13.36	4	36	5.75
Urban	136	19.97	5 or more	19	3.04
Suburban/rural	454	66.67			

preferences for *direct experience* and graphic, pictorial (*iconics*) modes of presentation would seem to support the supposition about the structure preference. Both of these modes involve active learning, which may help people with narcolepsy maintain attention in learning situations.

Relative to preferences for structure and the direct experience and iconics modes, preferences for *listening*, *reading*, and *affiliation* are significantly lower, but do not differ from each other. Since listening and reading are relatively passive learning modes, these lower preferences appear to be consistent with the difficulties narcoleptics report concerning learning. In passive learning situations people may experience more difficulty with maintaining attention and encoding information in memory. Lower preferences for affiliation indicate less interest in interpersonal contact with the instruc-

Table 2. Educational Background

Variable	N	%	Variable	N	%
Level of Education			**Major Narcolepsy**		
Elementary	17	2.49	**Information Source**		
Attended H.S.	59	8.65	MD	206	36.14
H.S. Diploma/equiv.	288	33.43	RN	3	.53
Attended College	187	27.42	Other Health		
Graduate 4 yr.			Provider	1	.18
College	191	28.01	Classes	5	.88
			Read	355	62.23
Yrs. since Graduation					
5 yrs. or less	100	14.99	**Time since Narcolepsy**		
6-10 yrs.	72	10.79	**Information**		
11-15 yrs.	54	8.10	Within month	107	16.02
16-20 yrs.	44	6.60	Within year	193	28.89
20 yrs. or more	397	59.52	2-3 years	99	14.82
			4-5 years	45	6.74
Participate in Learning			6 years or more	224	33.53
Classes					
Yes	565	82.97			
No	116	17.03			
Time since Learning					
Classes					
Regular attend					
every month	60	9.95			
Attend 3-4 times/					
yrs.	121	20.07			
1-2 yrs. since					
attend	122	20.23			
3-4 yrs. since					
attend	61	10.12			
5 yrs. or more					
since attend	239	39.64			

tor and peers during teaching-learning situations. In light of the lower preferences for affiliation, group education situations may be less effective with narcoleptic learners.

Preference for *achievement* is significantly lower than all of the modes as well as the structure and affiliation conditions. In terms of health education, people with narcolepsy may feel it is inappropriate to set their own goals or learn independently, especially when information obtained about this disorder from health care professionals can be crucial to achieving good symptom control and health maintenance. *Eminence* was significantly lower than all the other learning preferences. Authoritative, competitive learning situations may be counterproductive. People with narcolepsy may al-

FIGURE 3. Mean Learning Style Scale Scores

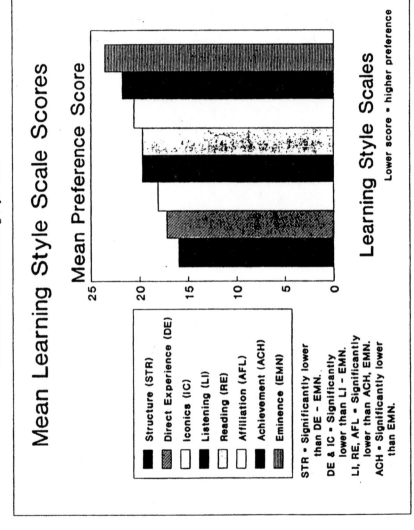

Mean Learning Style Scale Scores

Mean Preference Score

Structure (STR)
Direct Experience (DE)
Iconics (IC)
Listening (LI)
Reading (RE)
Affiliation (AFL)
Achievement (ACH)
Eminence (EMN)

STR - Significantly lower
    than DE - EMN.
DE & IC - Significantly
    lower than LI - EMN.
LI, RE, AFL - Significantly
    lower than ACH, EMN.
ACH - Significantly lower
    than EMN.

Learning Style Scales

Lower score = higher preference

ready lack confidence in their learning ability, and competitive learning situations could be further discouraging to these learners.

Stepwise multiple linear regression procedures revealed that some of the independent measures differentially accounted for variations in the learning style preference scores.

Significant predictors for the learning style scale scores and the amount of variation (R^2) accounted for by personal characteristics, narcolepsy symptoms, depression, and/or right/left motor and thinking patterns were as follows:

1. Affiliation — education, occupation, income, other symptoms, laterality, R^2 .085;
2. Structure — education, occupation, other symptoms, R/L thinking, R^2 .077;
3. Achievement — education, other symptoms, R^2 .041;
4. Eminence — education, new classic symptoms, R/L thinking, R^2 .096;
5. Listening — age, sex, new classic symptoms, depression, R^2 .036;
6. Reading — sex, new classic and learning and memory symptoms, laterality, R/L thinking, R^2 .065;
7. Direct Experience — new classic symptoms, R^2 .033.

None of the independent measures entered the regression equation for the iconics learning style scale score. In light of the memory and learning complaints of people with narcolepsy, it is somewhat surprising that this symptom score was a significant predictor for only one of the learning style scale scores. Overall selected personal characteristics were better predictors of learning style preference scores than the other independent measures. However, the evidence provided by the narcolepsy respondents was not substantial since the amount of variation explained was relatively small. Further research is needed into the reasons for learning style preference variations of people with narcolepsy.

CONCLUSION

The national sample of people with narcolepsy who participated in this study prefer structured teaching-learning situations that use the active learning modes of direct experience and graphic, pictorial (iconics) means of presentation. These preferences seem consistent with the complaints people with this disorder express relative to the concentration and memory difficulties they experience in attempting to learn new information. Underlying these preferences may be specific behavioral coping strategies that are being used to counteract sleepiness and decreases in attention span. More research is needed to examine the specific coping behaviors used, and their relationship to preferred learning style, as well as which factors are significant predictors of learning style preferences for people with narcolepsy.

REFERENCES

Aguirre, M., R. Broughton and D. Stuss. 1985. "Does Memory Impairment Exist in Narcolepsy-Cataplexy?" *Journal of Clinical and Experimental Neuropsychology* 7:14-24.

Briggs, G. C. and R. D. Nebes. 1975. "Patterns of Hand Preference in a Student Population." *Cortex* 11:230-238.

Broughton, R. and Q. Ghanem. 1976. "The Impact of Compound Narcolepsy on the Life of the Patient." In C. Guilleminault, W. C. Dement, and P. Passouant, eds. *Narcolepsy: Advances in Sleep Research*. New York: Spectrum, pp. 201-219.

Canfield, A. A. 1980. *Learning Styles Inventory Manual* (2nd ed.). Ann Arbor, MI: Humanics Medica.

Canfield, A. A. 1988. *Learning Styles Inventory Manual* (3rd ed.). Los Angeles, CA: Western Psychological Association.

Cohen, F. L. 1988. "Narcolepsy: A Review of a Common, Life-long Sleep Disorder." *Journal of Advanced Nursing* 13:546-556.

Crane, L. No date. *ALERT Scale of Thinking and Doing*. Western Michigan State University.

Kales, A., C. R. Soldatos, E. O. Bixler, A. Caldwell, R. J. Cadieux, J. M. Verrechio, and J. D. Kales. 1982. "Narcolepsy-Cataplexy: II. Psychological Consequences and Associated Psychopathology." *Archives of Neurology* 39:169-171.

Merritt, S. L. In press. "Learning Style Preferences of Coronary Artery Disease Patients." *Cardiovascular Nursing*.

Merritt, S. L. 1989. "Learning Styles: Theory and Use as a Basis for Instruction." In W. L. Holzemer, ed. *Review of Research in Nursing Education* vol. II. New York: National League for Nursing, pp. 1-31.

Merritt, S. L. and J. C. Marshall. 1984. "Reliability and Construct Validity of Alternate Forms of the CLS Inventory." *Advances in Nursing Science* 7, 78-85.

Messick, S. 1984. "The Nature of Cognitive Styles: Problems and Promise in Educational Practice." *Educational Psychologist* 19:59-74.

Rogers, A. E. and R. S. Rosenberg. 1990. "Tests of Memory in Narcoleptics." *Sleep* 13:42-52.

Rogers, A. E. 1984. "Problems and Coping Strategies Identified by Narcoleptic Patients." *J. of Neurosurgical Nursing* 16:326-334.

ADDITIONAL READING

Radloff, L. S. 1977. "The CES-D Scale: A Self-Report Depression Scale for Research in the General Population." *Journal of Applied Psychological Measurement* 1:385-401.

Radloff, L. S. and Locke, B. T. 1986. "The Community Mental Health Assessment Survey and the CES-D Scale." In M. M. Weissmann, J. K. Myers and C. E. Ross, eds. *Community Surveys of Psychiatric Disorders*. New York: Rutgers University Press, pp. 177-189.

SECTION III:
ISSUES IN THE MANAGEMENT OF NARCOLEPSY

The Realpolitik of Narcolepsy and Other Disorders with Impaired Alertness

Merrill M. Mitler

Man has generally expressed a mixed regard for sleep in our culture. While our literature recognizes sleep as a process that "knits the ravell'd sleave of care," humans have also expressed concern about mortal and morbid events during the night since recorded history. The Bible states that Solomon's bed was guarded by sixty valiant men throughout the night for fear of death (Song of Solomon 3:7-8). Virgil referred to sleep as "the kinsman of death" (The Aneid). In the 16th Century, St. John of the Cross referred to this issue in The Ascent of Mount Carmel (circa: 1578-1580). In mod-

Merrill M. Mitler, PhD, ACP,, is Director of Research, Sleep Disorders Center, Division of Chest Medicine, Critical Care and Sleep Disorders, Scripps Clinic and Research Foundation, La Jolla, CA.

Dr. Mitler is supported by NINDS grant RO1 NS20459 and a grant from the American Narcolepsy Association.

ern times, F. Scott Fitzgerald (1945) wrote: "In the real dark night of the soul it is always three o'clock in the morning." Ray Bradbury (1962) used the term "the soul's midnight" to refer to the clocktime, 3 a.m. There is some scientific justification for such concerns. Medical statistics dating to the late 1800's indicate that human mortality does rise rapidly from a low at 12 midnight-2 a.m. to a peak at 6-8 a.m. (von Jenny 1933).

SLEEP TENDENCY

In the past 15 years, the growth of research on sleep and the biological clocks that control it has led to significant discoveries about the many ways in which these processes influence human health and functioning (Association of Sleep Disorders Centers 1979; Moore-Ede et al. 1982; American Medical Association 1984). One is often unaware of these influences, which have a more profound effect than is generally realized. Research on the psychophysiology, neurophysiology, endocrinology, and behavioral aspects of disturbed and inappropriately timed sleep has led to a better understanding of the consequences of sleep disorders, improper sleep schedules, shiftwork, and daytime sleepiness.

One major discovery has been that the neural processes controlling alertness and sleep produce an increased sleep tendency and diminished capacity to function during certain early morning hours (circa 2-7 a.m.) and to a lesser degree during a period in the midafternoon (circa 2-5 p.m.), whether or not one has slept. (For a detailed review, see Mitler et al. 1988.) The data for Figure 1 are taken from the reports of the Stanford group under Carskadon (Dement and Carskadon 1982; Richardson et al. 1982). The figure represents the temporal distribution of unintended sleep episodes in a group of elderly people who were told to stay awake. The two-peak pattern in biological sleep tendency is clearly revealed by such studies. The pattern of increasing, then decreasing, sleepiness from noon to 8 p.m. has been widely replicated in clinical studies on control subjects and patients with sleep disorders using the Multiple Sleep Latency Test (Richardson et al. 1978) and the Maintenance of Wakefulness Test (Miller et al. 1982).

Other aspects of sleep, such as the stages of sleep obtained at

FIGURE 1. The temporal distribution of 278 unintended sleep episodes from the studies of Carskadon and colleagues (1981, 1982). The pattern from noon to 8 p.m. has been widely replicated in studies using the Multiple Sleep Latency Test and the Maintenance of Wakefulness Test.

SLEEPINESS

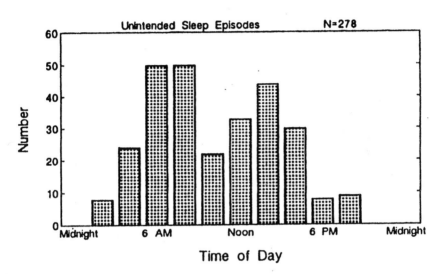

different times of day (Broughton 1975; Gagnon et al. 1985; Lavie, Wollman and Pollack 1986) and the frequency of naps (Dinges et al. 1980) also reveal a pattern of greater sleep pressure during these two time spans. Sleep and sleep-related processes can be linked to many aspects of human functioning ranging from automobile driver error (Langlois et al. 1985; Lavie, Wollman, and Pollack 1986) to disease-related mortality (Mitler and Kripke 1986; Mitler et al. 1987).

Superimposed on the normal, two-peak pattern of sleep vulnerability are the effects of two separate but interacting factors: (a) sleep deprivation, such as that occurring during accommodation to an unusual work schedule (Carskadon and Dement 1981) and (b) sleep disruption, such as that resulting from a sleep disorder (Carskadon, Brown and Dement 1982). Data from our field indicate that the effects of such sleep loss are cumulative. Thus, people who determine public policy and are responsible for risk management must appreciate that the danger of an error due to sudden overwhelming sleepiness increases progressively with continued sleep loss or "sleep debt." Most individuals cope with significant sleep debt by physical activity and dietary stimulants. Coping mechanisms can temporarily make an individual completely unaware of a dangerous accumulated sleep loss. But when defenses are "let down," such as during a period requiring immobility, overwhelming sleepiness ensues. Such unawareness may account for seemingly incomprehensible instances in which individuals have permitted themselves to sleep in circumstances that cause great hazard for themselves and others. Thus, the more sleep is disturbed or reduced, for whatever reason, the more likely an individual will inadvertently slip into sleep. There is laboratory evidence to suggest that even brief episodes of sleep, called "microsleeps," produce inattention, forgetfulness, and performance lapses, particularly during the two zones of vulnerability within the 24-hour cycle (Dinges 1988).

HUMAN MORTALITY

Our studies at Scripps Clinic and Research Foundation have confirmed and extended studies demonstrating that there is also a similar two-peak pattern throughout the 24-hour day in disease-related mortality. We found a 60% rise in human mortality from a low at about 2 a.m. to a high at about 8 a.m. (Mitler and Kripke 1986; Mitler et al. 1987). In addition, there is a smaller peak in the midafternoon at about 2 p.m.

Figure 2 presents the distribution about the 24-hours of disease-related mortalities taken collectively from Smolensky, Hallberg and Sargent (1972) and Mitler et al. (1987). Most of these mortalities have been attributed on the death certificates to ischemic heart disease. With respect to cardiac morbidity, rather than mortality, there is a similar two-peak curve. The Holter monitoring work of Araki et al. (1983) and Muller et al. (1985) on enzyme level confirmations of both lethal and nonlethal heart attack indicates a very clear two-peak pattern and further substantiates that the pattern is not due to some artifact of discovery or health care.

The work of Motta and Guilleminault (1985) on REM sleep-related cardiac arrhythmias, Timms et al. (1988) on respiration during

FIGURE 2. Temporal distribution of 437,511 human mortalities combined from the death certificate data of Smolensky, Halberg, and Sargent (1972) and Mitler et al. (1987).

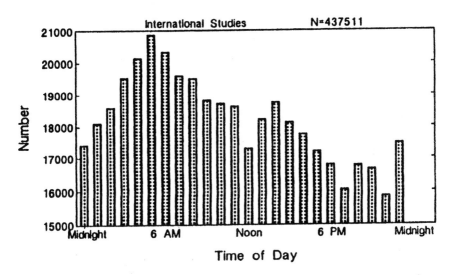

HUMAN MORTALITY

sleep in chronic obstructive pulmonary disease, and Mitler et al. (1988) on respiration during sleep after ethanol consumption all implicate sleep-specific physiological conditions in the elaboration of the two-peak pattern of disease-related mortality and morbidity.

In a review of literature on the biological tendency over the 24-hour day for mortality, for sleep, and for human error accidents, a committee of experts concluded that the separate two-peak curves generally have the same timing and shape (Mitler et al. 1988).

HUMAN ERROR

A number of evaluations have been conducted on vehicular accidents throughout the 24-hour day. Many factors can contribute to accidents, including road conditions, traffic congestion, and speed limits. Also, the total number of automobile and truck accidents is generally greater during the daytime hours (circa 10 a.m.-6 p.m.)

than at other times because of increased vehicle traffic during this time (Duff, unpublished; Langlois et al. 1985; Lavie, Wollman and Pollak 1986). Of special interest is the temporal distribution of single-vehicle accidents (e.g., driving off the road), because it is suspected that these accidents have a greater probability of being related to inadvertent lapses in driver attention.

Studies of single-vehicle automobile accidents reveal a bimodal temporal pattern. Figure 3 presents the temporal distribution of 6,052 single-vehicle traffic accidents attributed to "falling asleep at the wheel" taken from studies in New York (Duff unpublished), Texas (Langlois et al. 1985), and Israel (Lavie, Wollman and Pollak 1986). The major peak is between midnight and 7 a.m. and is especially pronounced between 1 and 4 a.m. A small secondary peak is visible between 1 and 4 p.m. When the incidence among various age groups is examined, this secondary peak becomes more pronounced in drivers over 45 years of age (Langlois et al. 1985).

FIGURE 3. Temporal distribution of 6,052 vehicular accidents that were judged by investigators to be fatigue-related, displayed as a function of time of day. The figure combines the samples of Lavie, Wollman, and Pollack (Israel: N = 390); Langlois et al. (Texas: N = 4,994) and Duff (New York: N = 668).

FATIGUE-RELATED TRAFFIC ACCIDENTS

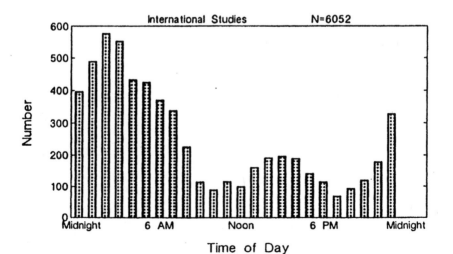

All other vehicle accident data available appear to be consistent with the temporal distribution depicted in Figure 2 (Hildebrandt, Rehmert and Rutenfranz 1974; Mackie and Miller 1978; Pokorny, Blom, and Van Leewan 1981a, 1981b; Prokop and Prokop 1955).

Thus extensive data from disparate fields indicate that there is a two-peak curve not only in susceptibility to sleep, but also in susceptibility to mortality and to error. I submit that these curves all reflect some underlying process that is a fundamental property of the human condition.

SHIFTWORK

People involved in shiftwork planning have been among the first to make use of the data from our field of sleep research in shiftwork planning. Those involved in round-the-clock operations recognize that there are limitations in the capacity of human sleep-wake cycles to adjust to changes in rotating work schedules.

Evening and night work disrupts the normal human sleep-wakefulness cycle, creating problems that take many different forms. In general, shiftwork can present three major biological problems to workers. First, work is often performed during the trough in the circadian rhythm of alertness. Second, desynchronization of the body's circadian rhythms leads to pervasive feelings of fatigue and malaise ("occupational jet lag"). Third, disruption of sleep-wake cycles results in accumulated sleep deficit toward the end of a shift series.

The consequences of shiftwork manifest themselves in a variety of ways. Approximately 20% of shiftworkers experience gastrointestinal disorders. Disruptions of their social and family lives compound the physical stress of these work schedules on the human body. Sleep-deprived shiftworkers often experience involuntary lapses of attention halfway between sleep and wakefulness: they may appear to be awake as they perform routine tasks, yet they are impaired in their responses to unanticipated stimuli (e.g., warning signals). Frequently, these workers make serious errors which can contribute to or cause accidents. In field studies of 1500 workers in a dozen industrial sites, over 55% of the workers admitted to "nodding off" or falling asleep on the job during a given week.

Despite these problems of shiftwork, the demands of modern society require that we rely upon workers day and night to remain vigilant while operating complex machinery or while performing repetitive production line tasks. Major investments by industry in capital equipment, and the services of police, fire, and medical personnel, all demand continuous round-the-clock operation. In fact, shiftwork in technologically advanced nations has grown dramatically in the past 20 years; approximately one-third of the U.S. labor force works a rotating schedule (Mitler et al. 1988).

These data underscore the importance of medical evaluation of people who complain that they cannot stay awake. There are several etiologically distinct disorders that give rise to the symptom of excessive somnolence. For example, narcolepsy is a genetic neurological disorder linked to the human leukocyte antigen phenotype DR2 (Matsuki et al. 1985; Mitler et al. 1986) that best responds to stimulant drugs such as methylphenidate and pemoline. Sleep apnea syndrome is linked to anatomically abnormal narrowing of the upper airway that best responds to surgical revision or mechanical airway support (Strohl, Cherniak and Gothe 1986).

The largest segment of the somnolent patient population is diagnosed as having sleep apnea. The presence of a sleep disorder characterized by the symptom of excessive somnolence is not thought to alter the underlying mechanisms that schedule sleep within the body. Rather, such disorders change the set point for sleep, i.e., raise the baseline of sleep tendency. George et al. (1987) and Findley, Unversagt and Surrat (1988) have shown that sleep apnea patients are seven times more likely to have automobile accidents than control subjects. Thus, such somnolent patients are more likely to contribute to the accident statistics, but are not likely to change the temporal distribution of accidents. Other major diagnostic groups with the symptom of somnolence are narcolepsy, sleep deprivation (with and without alcohol involvement), and misuse of sleeping pills. Patients in these diagnostic entities experience daytime sleepiness that can reach disabling levels of severity. However, even with greatly increased overall tendency to sleep, the two-peak pattern in physiologic sleep tendency is maintained throughout the 24-hour day — the baseline is simply elevated. This point cannot be over-emphasized in the context of problems with shiftwork.

CIRCADIAN CONTROL

The circadian timing system is centered deep within the hypothalamus above the optic chiasm in the suprachiasmatic nucleus (Moore-Ede, Sulzman and Fuller 1982). This mechanism has two functions: to keep us properly timed to the day-night cycle of our environment, and to synchronize various functions of the body. The human body is "programmed" in time to coordinate behavior with the time of day. Most physiological functions perform at maximum efficiency during the daytime when people working traditional jobs need to be most alert. However, workers on rotating shifts need to perform during nontraditional work hours and at times when the body is geared toward sleep.

Based upon numerous laboratory and field studies, it has been found that the human body generally runs on a 25-hour cycle, or one hour longer than the earth's day-night cycle. As a result, the body is easily capable of resetting the internal clock by an hour each day, if the new schedule is later than the previous one. Many work schedules, however, require workers to jump from shift to shift on a weekly basis, often in a backwards direction (each new shift being eight hours earlier). As a result, this drastic resetting of the internal clock may take three days to a week to accomplish.

RISK MANAGEMENT

Management's prime goal in designing rotating shiftwork schedules should be to alleviate the biological problems listed above. A properly designed schedule will not only enhance worker health and satisfaction, but can bring about major improvements in health, safety, and productivity as well. Experiments carried out by the Center for the Design of Industrial Schedules (CDIS), a nonprofit service organization affiliated with Harvard University, have provided significant research results in this area and demonstrated the effectiveness of improved shift schedule designs.

In 1983 the Philadelphia police officer's union invited the CDIS, under the supervision of Dr. Charles Czeisler of Harvard University, to create a schedule that would better serve the needs of both the officers and their commanders. Dissatisfaction among patrolmen on the "old" schedule was high; three-quarters of the officers were willing to try whatever schedule the CDIS group developed. The old schedule required six days of work in a row before receiving two days off; the next new shift was eight hours earlier. Evaluation of the old schedule revealed the following: (1) Over 50% of the officers reported a moderate to severe problem with poor quality sleep; (2) On the night shift, almost 80% of the officers fell asleep at least once during a week; (3) One-quarter of the officers reported being involved in an actual or near-miss automobile accident due to on-the-job sleepiness during the past year; (4) Night shift officers drank heavily, compared with day workers and other shiftworkers; (5) Over 75% of officers' families were dissatisfied with their work schedules; (6) Thirty-five percent of the officers took either an entire week to adjust or never adjusted to the weekly shift rotation.

After evaluating the old schedule, the CDIS recommended an improved schedule that included the following characteristics: (1) The direction of rotation was changed from backward (day to night to afternoon shift) to forward (day to afternoon to night shift); (2) The rate of rotation was reduced from one week to three weeks; (3) The six-day work week was reduced to four or five work days in a row; (4) Staffing levels were designed to reflect demands for police coverage, which varied throughout the day.

In December 1986, after an 11-month trial period, the improved schedule was evaluated in comparison to the old schedule. Some noteworthy results include: (1) Officers reported a four-fold decrease in the frequency of poor sleep; (2) Officers reported a 25% decline in the number of sleep episodes on the night shift; (3) Officers had 40% fewer on-the-job automobile accidents per mile driven; (4) Officers used fewer sleeping pills and less alcohol to alleviate the consequences of sleep deprivation; (5) Officers' families reported a nearly five-fold increase in satisfaction with their work schedule; (6) Twice as many officers preferred the improved schedule over the old schedule.

It is important to note that, in the face of these results, management and labor were nevertheless unable to agree on implementation of a biologically-sound revision of the Philadelphia Police Department's work schedule. In fact, as a punitive step, the widely-preferred experimental schedule was cancelled. This situation underscores the necessity for better management-labor cooperation on biological needs of shiftworkers. It is often not enough to work out a scientifically sound work schedule. It is also necessary to have all parties treat the new schedule as a "biologically mandated given" and not as a management-labor "bargaining chip."

This kind of cooperation requires real effort. Workers often value extended time off and freedom to work a second job more than they value reduction in accidents and increases in productivity. It is necessary to appeal to the "significant players" in shiftwork scheduling on grounds that are relevant to their own agendas. For example, management may be persuaded by improved risk management and worker productivity. On the other hand, labor may be persuaded by increased job safety and fewer health problems for workers. Regulatory agencies are also often involved and may be persuaded by improved public safety and reduced risks of environmental catastrophes.

Thus, although few managers, workers, or government regulators would argue against the need for, say, clean drinking water in the workplace, many do not support the unequivocal need for work schedules that have been shown to improve the performance and the overall health of shiftworkers.

MATHEMATICAL MODEL

Although the two-peak pattern in our temporal existence is apparent from a great variety of studies, current circadian rhythms theory has not produced testable models of the two-peak pattern in human performance and sleep tendency throughout the 24-hour day.

I propose the following mathematical model for consideration:

Equation 1.

$$P = 1/K \left[K - (COS^2(t + phi)) (1 - COS(t + phi) / SD)^2 \right]$$

Where P   =   Performance
       K   =   Scaler
       t   =   Clock time
       phi =   Physiological phase offset
       SD =   Sleep Deprivation factor

A mirror image of the curve that is useful for modeling sleep tendency is given by:

Equation 2.

$$S = 1 - (1/K [K - (COS^2(t + phi)) (1 - COS(t + phi) / SD)^2])$$

This function is plotted in Figure 4.

Both equation 1 and equation 2 are essentially amalgamations of the familiar cosine function that has been traditionally used to describe circadian functions and an equation often used to predict fluctuations in the populations of various species:

$$P_{n+1} = rP_n(1 - P_n)$$

In this equation, P represents population size and r is a growth rate parameter. The equation has also been much studied with respect to the value of r by those interested in the field of chaos.

The correlation between actual numbers of over 437,000 human deaths throughout the 24 hours and predicted values is 0.70 ($p < .0005$), the equation accounting for 49% of the variance. For over 6000 fatigue-related auto accidents, the correlation between observed and predicted hourly values is 0.80 ($p < .0005$), the equation accounting for 65% of the variance. The three curves are superimposed in Figure 5.

I suggest that the predictive power of the cosine-population function derives from both circadian factors and from fluctuations in sleep tenency that depend on actual numbers of receptor populations in the brain that are important for the behavioral expression of sleep. I encourage further testing and refinement of the equation by all who have appropriate data.

PRESCRIPTIONS FOR THE FUTURE

A recent inquiry in the United States found that a major railroad accident in Pennsylvania, was caused by train crew falling asleep at the controls (Conrail, based in Connecticut). Here is yet another human error accident resulting in multiple deaths. Similar kinds of errors may be at the root of the recent British Rail accidents. The

FIGURE 4. Double plot (48-hour) of the function in Equation 2 that is taken to represent sleep tendency. For this particular curve K = 1.8, SD = 3 and phi = 120.

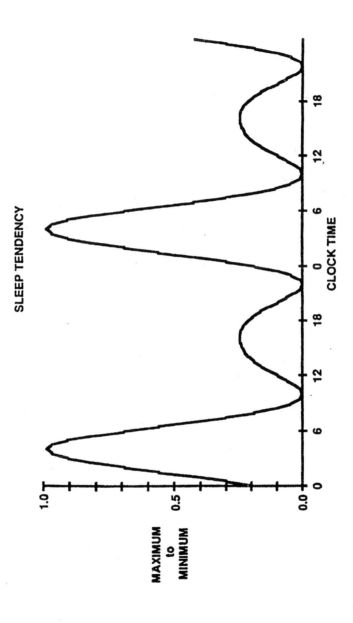

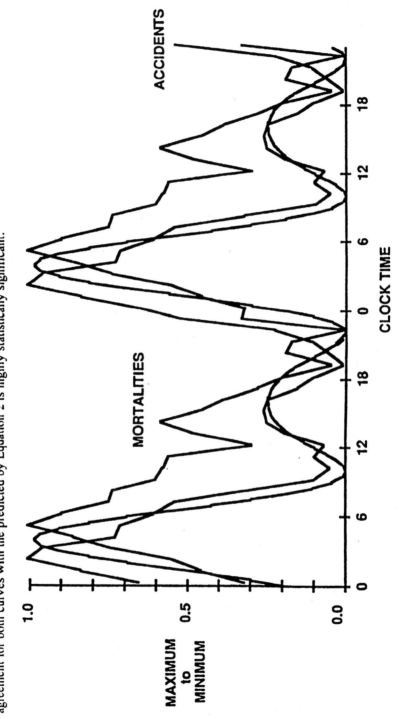

FIGURE 5. Double plots of the mirror image of Equation 1 that is given by Equation 2 along with the human mortality data of Figure 2 and the automobile accident data of Figure 3. Note that the human mortality has a higher afternoon peak than the accidents. However, the agreement for both curves with the predicted by Equation 2 is highly statistically significant.

list of human error accidents—Chernobyl, Three Mile Island and others—continues to grow alarmingly.

The prevailing public reaction to such accidents goes something like this: People don't care any more about doing their job right. They use drugs, they drink, they fall asleep. We should get tougher. But this reaction is wrong and counterproductive; we should really get kinder and gentler.

People fall asleep according to biological laws and have been doing so since prehistoric times—often while at work. What is really worrisome is that so many more people can be hurt when a train driver or a nuclear power engineer falls asleep in 1989, than when, say, a stagecoach driver fell asleep in 1889. The chances of someone sleeping on the job have not changed. Rather, it is the costs in life and property of such sleeping that have changed. Risk management must intelligently accommodate to these new costs. For example, workers must be selected for their ability to stay awake, not for their willingness to work nights. Some recommendations for consideration are:

- Risks due to sleep are so much greater now than 50-100 years ago, that fundamentally different approaches are required for risk management;
- Work-rest schedules for industries that operate round the clock must be biologically compatible with human sleep requirements;
- Drivers, particularly those who transport the public or dangerous materials, should be regularly tested for their ability to stay awake on the job;
- People with sleep pathologies such as sleep apnea and narcolepsy must be rapidly identified and treated;
- National governments, because of delays that stem from management-labor negotiations, must take the lead in formulating new hiring and scheduling guidelines that do not place workers at jobs and schedules for which they are biologically unsuited;
- Just as the major industrial nations have recently decided to act on, rather than talk about, reductions in chlorofleurocarbons, these countries must also act to reduce dangers of sleeping on the job; .

We now have the knowledge and know-how to respond to the clear and present dangers of sleeping on the job. Do we really need a Chernobyl or a Bhopal to get going?

REFERENCES

American Medical Association. 1984. *Guide to Better Sleep*. New York: Random House.

Araki, H., Y. Koiwaya, O. Nakagaki et al. 1983. "Diurnal Distribution of ST-segment Elevation and Related Arrhythmias in Patients with Variant Angina: A Study by Ambulatory ECG Monitoring." *Circulation* 67:995-1000.

Association of Sleep Disorders Centers. 1979. "Diagnostic Classification of Sleep and Arousal Disorders, First Edition," prepared by the Sleep Disorders Classification Committee. *Sleep* 2:1-137.

Bradbury, R. 1962. *Something Wicked This Way Comes*. Englewood Cliffs, NJ: Simon and Schuster.

Broughton, R. 1975. "Biorhythmic Variations in Consciousness and Psychological Functions." *Canadian Psychological Review* 16:217-239.

Carskadon, M. A., E. D. Brown, and W. C. Dement. 1982. "Sleep Fragmentation in the Elderly: Relation to Daytime Sleep Tendency." *Neurobiology of Aging* 3:321-327.

Carskadon, M. A. and W. C. Dement. 1981. "Cumulative Effects of Sleep Restriction on Daytime Sleepiness." *Psychophysiology* 18:107-113.

Dement, W. C. and M. A. Carskadon. 1982. "An Essay on Sleepiness." In M. Baldy-Moulinier, ed. *Actualités en Medicine Expérimentale: En Homage au Professeur P. Passouant*. Montpelier: Euromed, pp. 46-71.

Dinges, D. F. 1988. "The Nature of Sleepiness: Causes, Contexts and Consequences." In A. Baum and A. Stunkard, eds. *Perspectives in Behavioral Medicine*. NJ: Erlbaum.

Dinges, D. F., M. T. Orne, and F. J. Evans. 1980. "Voluntary Self-Control of Sleep to Facilitate Quasi-Continuous Performance." In *U.S. Army Medical Research and Development Command Report No. 80*, U.S. Army Medical Research and Development Command, Fort Detrick, Frederick, MD.

Findley, L. J., M. E. Unverzagt, and P. M. Suratt. 1988. "Automobile Accidents Involving Patients with Obstructive Sleep Apnea. *American Review of Respiratory Disorders* 138:337-340.

Fitzgerald, F. S. 1945. "The Crack-up." In E. Wilson, ed. *The Hours*. New York: John Peale Bishop.

Gagnon, P., J. De Konick, and R. Broughton. 1985. "Reappearance of Electroencephalogram Slow Waves in Extended Sleep with Delayed Bedtime." *Sleep* 8:18-128.

George, C. F., P. W. Nickerson, P. J. Hanley et al. 1987. "Sleep Apnea Patients Have More Automobile Accidents" [letter]. *Lancet* 2:447.

Hildebrandt, G., W. Rehmert, and J. Rutenfranz. 1974. "Twelve- and Twenty-

Four-Hour Rhythms in Error Frequency of Locomotive Drivers and the Influence of Tiredness." *International Journal of Chronobiology* 2:175-180.

Langlois, P. H., M. H. Smolensky, B. P. Hsi et al. 1985. "Temporal Patterns of Reported Single-Vehicle Car and Truck Accidents in Texas, U.S.A. During 1980-1983." *Chronobiology International* 2:131-140.

Lavie, P., M. Wollman, and I. Pollack. 1986. "Frequency of Sleep-Related Traffic Accidents and Hour of the Day." *Sleep Research* 15:275.

Mackie, R. R. and J. C. Miller. 1978. "Effects of Hours of Service, Regularity of Schedules, and Cargo Loading on Truck and Bus Driver Fatigue." Human Factors Research, Inc. Technical Report No. 1765-F, Washington, DC, Department of Transportation, Bureau of Motor Carrier Safety, FHWA and National Highway Traffic Safety Administration.

Matsuki, K., T. Juji, K. Tokunaga et al. 1985. "Human Histocompatibility Leukocyte Antigen (HLA) Haplotype Frequencies Estimated from the Data on HLA Class I, II, and III Antigens in 111 Japanese Narcoleptics." *Journal of Clinical Investigation* 76:2078-2083.

Mitler, M. M., Czeisler, C. A., Carskadon, M. A. et al. 1988. "Sleep, Catastrophes and Public Policy." *Sleep* 11:100-109.

Mitler, M., K. Gujavarty, and C. Browman. 1982. "Maintenance of Wakefulness Test: A Polysomnographic Technique for Evaluating Treatment in Patients with Excessive Somnolence." *Electroencephalograph Clinical Neurophysiology* 53:658-661.

Mitler, M. M., R. M. Hajdukovich, R. Shafor et al. 1987. "When People Die: Causes of Death Versus Time of Death." *American Journal of Medicine* 82:266-274.

Mitler, M. M. and D. F. Kripke. 1986. "Circadian Variation in Myocardial Infarction." *New England Journal of Medicine* 314:1187-1188.

Mitler, M. M., A. Dawson, S. J. Henriksen, M. Sobers, and F. E. Bloom. 1988. "Bedtime Ethanol Increases Upper Airways Resistance and Produces Sleep Apneas in Asymptomatic Snorers." *Alcoholism: Clinical and Experimental Research* 12:801-805.

Moore-Ede, M. C., F. M. Sulzman, and C. A. Fuller. 1982. *The Clocks that Time Us.* Cambridge, MA: Harvard University Press.

Motta, J. and C. Guilleminault. 1985. "Cardiac Dysfunction During Sleep." *Annals of Clinical Research* 17:190-198.

Muller, J. E., P. H. Stone, Z. G. Turi et al. 1985. "Circadian Variation in the Frequency of Onset of Acute Myocardial Infarction." *New England Journal of Medicine* 313:1315-1322.

Pokorny, M. L. I., D. H. J. Blom, and P. van Leewan. 1981a. "Analysis of Traffic Accident Data (from Bus Drivers): An Alternative Approach (I)." In A. Reinberg, N. Viex, and P. Andlauer, eds. *Night and Shift Work: Biological and Social Aspects.* New York: Pergamon Press.

Pokorny, M. L. I., D. H. J. Blom, and P. van Leewan. 1981b. "Analysis of Traffic Accident Data (from Bus Drivers): An Alternative Approach (II)." In

A. Reinberg, N. Viex, and P. Andlauer, eds. *Night and Shift Work: Biological and Social Aspects*. New York: Pergamon Press.

Prokop, O. and L. Prokop. 1955. "Ermudung und Einschlafen am Steuer (Fatigue and Falling Asleep While Driving)." *Dtsch Z Gerichtl Med* 44:343-355.

Richardson, G., M. A. Carskadon, W. Flagg et al. 1978. "Excessive Daytime Sleepiness in Man: Multiple Sleep Latency Measurement in Narcoleptic and Control Subjects." *Electroencephalograph Clinical Neurophysiology* 45:621-627.

Richardson, G. S., M. A. Carskadon, E. J. Orav et al. 1982. "Circadian Variation of Sleep Tendency in Elderly and Young Adult Subjects." *Sleep* 5:S82-S84.

Smolensky, M., F. Halberg, and F. Sargent. 1972. "Chronobiology of the Life Sequence." In S. Ito, K. Ogata, and H. Yoshimura, eds. *Advances in Climatic Physiology*. Tokyo: Igaku Shoin, p. 281.

Strohl, K. P., N. S. Cherniack, and B. Gothe. 1986. "Physiologic Basis of Therapy for Sleep Apnea." *American Review of Respiratory Disorders* 134:791-802.

Timms, R. M., A. Dawson, R. M. Hajdukovic, M. M. Mitler. 1988. "Effect of Triazolam on Sleep and Arterial Oxygen Saturation in Patients with Chronic Obstructive Pulmonary Disease." *Archives of Internal Medicine* 148:2159-2163.

von Jenny, E. 1933. "Tagesperiodisch Einflusse auf Geburt und Tod." *Schweiz Med Wochenschr* 14:15-17.

ADDITIONAL READING

Carskadon, M. A. and W. C. Dement. 1982. "Nocturnal Determinants of Daytime Sleepiness." *Sleep* 5:S73-S81.

Mitler, M., J. van den Hoed, M. Carskadon et al. 1979. "REM Sleep Episodes During the Multiple Sleep Latency Test in Narcoleptic Patients." *Electroencephalograph Clinical Neurophysiology* 46:479-481.

Chronobiological Findings in Narcolepsy and Their Implications for Treatment and Psychosocial Adjustment

Charles P. Pollak

The cardinal and most disabling symptom of narcolepsy is the inability to stay awake and alert in the daytime (Rosenthal et al. in press). As a result, people with narcolepsy are globally impaired, often for much of the day and throughout their lifetimes (Broughton and Ghanem 1976). Because sleepiness is also experienced by non-narcoleptic people whenever their sleep is disrupted or shortened, the pathological nature of the narcoleptic sleep tendency is not always apparent to the affected person or family members. People with narcolepsy therefore delay seeking medical attention and, when they do, it is often with the ambition to eradicate any need to sleep in the daytime. Physicians often share this goal and prescribe high doses of stimulant drugs. Others with narcolepsy avoid medical care and simply try to hide the disorder. The impact of narco-

---

Charles P. Pollak, MD, is Head, Sleep/Wake Disorders Clinic, and Director, Institute of Chronobiology, New York Hospital-Cornell Medical Center, Westchester Division, White Plains, NY; also, he is Associate Professor of Neurology in Psychiatry and Neurology, Cornell University Medical College, New York, NY.

The author expresses his gratitude to colleagues D. Wagner, M. Moline, and J. Green, and to A. Stroud, K. Tucker, and other members of the Institute of Chronobiology for collecting and analyzing the voluminous data from each subject.

This research was supported by National Institute of Mental Health Grant PO1 MH37814 to C. P. Pollak.

Requests for reprints should be addressed to Charles Pollak, MD, Institute of Chronobiology, New York Hospital-Cornell Medical Center, Westchester Division, 21 Bloomingdale Road, White Plains, NY 10605.

lepsy therefore depends on the severity of the disorder, the effects of drugs and other countermeasures, occupational demands, personality, and social support or disapproval.

To measure the effects of proposed and established treatments, to assess the clinical effects of the psychosocial factors, and to provide rational counseling, it is necessary to disentangle these factors. The laboratory technique of temporal isolation offers a means of doing so. People with narcolepsy can be observed and monitored while they live in a laboratory setting where there are few social demands and no yardstick of time by which subjects can plan their activities. Initial findings from such studies have clarified several aspects of the physiology of narcolepsy, but this review will focus on their implications for medical management and especially for the psychosocial well-being of the person with narcolepsy.

METHOD

Six narcoleptic subjects and seven controls lived in one of four temporal isolation apartments maintained by the Institute of Chronobiology, New York Hospital-Cornell Medical Center. To deprive the subjects of a knowledge of time, the apartment had no windows, clocks, radio, or television. Technicians and other staff members entered the apartment frequently, but they worked shifts that were randomized with respect to both time of day and duration.

The diagnosis of narcolepsy was established by a detailed medical history that included the occurrence of cataplexy and a positive Multiple Sleep Latency Test (Carskadon et al. 1986; Mitler et al. 1979). The narcoleptic subjects and controls were in good general health and were drug-free for at least 14 days before entering the laboratory. They gave informed consent. Several narcoleptic subjects were motivated to participate by curiosity about their "natural" sleep patterns: would they sleep "all the time," for example?

Subjects were studied under two conditions, (1) entrainment of biological rhythms by a schedule and (2) free-running. During the first four to six laboratory days, subjects were asked to retire, to arise, and to eat meals on a 24-hour schedule. During the bed rest periods, room lights were extinguished. After completing the extrainment phase, the subjects were allowed to retire, arise, and eat whenever they chose ("free-running"). As during the entrained phase, room lights were extinguished whenever the subject was in bed. The absence of clocks meant that subjects could not pace their activities by anything except their own, inner sense of time.

Subjects were instructed not to sleep unless they were in bed in the darkness. Indeed, they were not allowed to lie down on the bed at other times. This was done to simulate the usual condition of everyday life in which opportunities for daytime sleep are narrowly restricted. It also assured us that any naps were involuntary. Naps were not interrupted, however, making it possible to measure their duration and sleep stage composition.

A broad range of variables was measured: rectal temperature, plasma cortisol and other hormones, sleep, eating behavior, subjective alertness, mood, and performance on several kinds of tasks. EEG, EOG, and EMG were continuously monitored from narcoleptic subjects, recorded on paper, and "scored" by the conventional method (Rechtschaffen and Kales 1968). Along with continuous observation by closed circuit television, this made it possible to detect all lapses of alertness and sleep episodes.

RESULTS

It quickly became apparent during the entrainment phase that the narcoleptic subjects differed from the controls. The narcoleptic subjects obtained most of their sleep during the bed rest periods; but none of the subjects was able to limit sleep to those periods. Every narcoleptic subject fell asleep repeatedly while seated in a chair during the "waking" day. When the narcoleptic subjects were allowed to free-run, they selected bed rest periods at normal, circadian intervals. Even then, despite having unrestricted periods for bed rest at circadian intervals, the narcoleptic subjects continued to nap. The naps occurred from 1.6 to 4.0 times a "day," lasted from 30.0 to 49.4 minutes, and accounted for 8.1-31.5% of total sleep time. By contrast, none of the controls was ever observed to nap.

The consistent, daily need of narcoleptic subjects to nap (i.e., to sleep at short intervals) may be explained in several ways. The first is loss of circadian control. It is well known that the sleep-wake pattern is normally governed by a circadian timing system (Wever

1979). If the signals from this system were weak, the circadian organization of sleep and waking periods would be partially lost. The daily waking period would contain episodes of sleep and the sleep period would contain episodes of wakefulness. The output of the circadian timing system is represented by the rhythms of core body temperature and plasma cortisol. These rhythms were found to be normal in the narcoleptic subjects, except for a low amplitude of body temperature in the oldest narcoleptic subject. As we have already seen, the periods of bed rest and darkness were also spaced at normal, circadian intervals. If the narcoleptic sleep pattern is not fully circadian, then, as indicated by "leaking" of sleep into the "waking" day in the form of naps, it is not because the circadian timing system is inactive. Perhaps it is not coupled normally to the brain mechanisms responsible for the states of sleep and wakefulness.

Another explanation of the need to nap is that the narcoleptic subjects were unable to get enough sleep during the bed rest periods. Restriction of the opportunity to sleep could be ruled out, since free-running subjects could spend as much time in bed as they chose. Also, they were able to utilize that time for sleep: sleep efficiency, total sleep time, and time spent in sleep stages 3, 4 and REM were similar to controls. The narcoleptic subjects did however, spend more time in light sleep (stage 1) and less in stage 2.

While the narcoleptic subjects obtained about as much deep sleep at night as the controls, there was the possibility that the narcoleptic subjects had an increased *need* for sleep that could not be filled at night. We found, however, that the fraction of time spent sleeping by the free-running narcoleptic subjects was not greater than that of the controls. Furthermore, the ability of the narcoleptic subjects to perform cognitive and motor tasks was only slightly impaired (Pollack, Moline, and Wagner 1990), and the mean level of subjective alertness did not decrease over the course of the experiment. The sleep obtained by them was therefore sufficient to prevent the effects expected from cumulative sleep loss (Pollak, Wagner, and Moline 1990). We infer that their total "need" for sleep was not increased, at least for the duration of the experiment. This was also true for sleep stages 3, 4, and REM.

It is worth observing that, since sleep duration was not increased, total waking time was not reduced. Because of the naps, however, waking time was not available as a single, daily block. Episodes of wakefulness lasted an average of 304 minutes.

Finally, we considered the possibility that the naps were triggered by another daytime event. The temporal pattern of naps was indeed found to be strongly correlated with that of meals. The frequency of naps increased about 1/2 hour after meal onset and then remained elevated for several hours. This increase of napping was not related to the size of the preceding meal and was therefore unlikely to be induced by the food itself. It may have been a preabsorptive effect of eating, such as gastroduodenal distention. Another possibility is that the increase of napping was an effect of a circadian timing mechanism. In several free-running, narcoleptic subjects, the circadian rhythm of meals was found to be synchronous with that of the bed rest periods, even when these rhythms were not synchronous with other circadian rhythms (Pollak and Green 1989). This has also been found in normal subjects (Aschoff et al. 1986; Green, Pollak, and Smith 1987) and suggests that meals and bed rest periods are timed by a common mechanism. The naps may have been an additional effect of that mechanism.

DISCUSSION

Our findings may be summarized as follows. The biological clock that governs sleep and wakefulness appears to function normally in subjects with narcolepsy. The subjects were able to use their inner sense of circadian time as cues for retiring and turning the lights off, followed by arising and turning them on. However, they were not able to confine sleep to the bed rest periods and slept at relatively short intervals. The mechanism underlying the narcoleptic nap has not been identified but may be a circadian clock. We now turn to the psychosocial implications of these findings.

Judging from their subjective ratings of alertness and their ability to perform a variety of tasks, the narcoleptic subjects were not very sleepy between naps. Therefore, sleepiness may not be intrinsic to narcolepsy. Since sleepiness is often present in the everyday lives of people with narcolepsy, however, it is time to consider whether it may be induced by interactions with the everyday physical and social environment. In particular, people attempting to live and work in a society that lives by the clock, including those with narcolepsy, simply cannot afford to nap. Since the naps are part of their daily sleep quota, however, success in suppressing them may induce sleep deprivation and result in intense sleepiness, sleep "attacks," and automatic behavior. Even cataplexy is reported to be increased at times of increased sleepiness. Time-isolation experiments employing strenuous suppression of naps will be required to demonstrate the adverse effects of suppressing naps.

Until such experiments have been carried out, it seems prudent to assume that strenuous suppression of naps can incur penalties that outweigh any advantages of avoiding daytime sleep. The usual aim of treatment—to eradicate all manifestations of narcolepsy, including naps—should therefore be replaced by a policy of *encouraging* naps. Such a policy offers the possibility that the subjective sleepiness, sleep "attacks," and automatic behavior associated with narcolepsy could be reduced or even eliminated. In addition, high doses of stimulant drugs might be avoided.

The optimal number and duration of naps appear to vary from person to person. Our data indicate that one to four naps a day lasting 30-50 minutes are needed by most affected individuals. For several reasons, therapeutic naps should be *scheduled*. First, to allow for regular naps, time slots for daytime sleep have to be created by scheduling competing daytime activities. This should ingrain the practice of napping and improve compliance. Second, the beneficial effects of sleep on subsequent periods of wakefulness are likely to be more predictable if naps occur at regular phases of the biological day. The person with narcolepsy can then better rely on himself or herself to maintain an expected level of alertness while performing a certain task at a certain time of day.

The burden of taking out time to nap may be lightened by recalling that our findings also show that total sleep need is not increased in narcolepsy. Aggregate waking time is therefore normal. If the available waking time can be put to productive use, people with narcolepsy can be as productive as those who sleep only once a day.

The disadvantages of therapeutic naps must also be recognized. These are primarily *psychosocial*. We in the United States live in a society that stigmatizes napping and provides almost no opportunities for it outside of schools for the very young. The urban centers where most people work are designed for commuting, making it impossible to return home to eat and sleep, as is often done in societies that have a siesta. The single daily work period lasts about 7 1/2 hours plus one or several hours for commuting. It therefore greatly outlasts the mean waking period of our narcoleptic subjects (304 minutes) and is broken by only a short lunch period and several "coffee breaks." These offer scant time for effective napping, not to speak of the lack of places to lie down and the disapproval of co-workers and employers.

For these reasons, the use of therapeutic naps should not be viewed as an alternative to drug therapy. Until social attitudes change, it is as unrealistic to expect to entirely replace stimulant drugs with naps as it may have been to expect drugs to eliminate the need to nap. We view therapeutic napping as an essential component of a multifaceted therapeutic program that also includes counseling, psychosocial support, modest daily doses of stimulants, and sometimes additional medications for control of the accessory symptoms of narcolepsy.

To counsel patients with narcolepsy effectively, we will need to rethink the types of work for which they are and are not suited. Our studies have shown that the person with narcolepsy is much less limited in *what* or *how much* can be done than in *when* and *for how long* it can be done. Jobs with long or unpredictable duty cycles are thus less suitable than those with short, self-paced periods of activity. For example, floor nursing can be a suitable occupation because a place and time to nap are sometimes provided. By contrast, assisting in lengthy surgical operations, sometimes at short notice, is a set-up for failure and danger.

Counseling must also address the personality and self-image of the person with narcolepsy. We have seen several self-employed narcoleptic people become disabled because they could not accept the need to take regular nap breaks. Fundamentally, they had not accepted the disorder as an ineradicable component of daily life. Accepting the diagnosis of narcolepsy is also a precondition for long-term compliance with medication regimens. Counseling should include family members, who must be taught to remind the affected person to nap and free the person of competing responsibilities at nap times.

Narcolepsy is one of a growing number of disorders for which education and long-term psychosocial support are as important as somatic treatments. Sleep disorders centers are the logical providers of these services, but not all of them do so. It is time they did.

REFERENCES

Aschoff, J., C., C. von Goetz, C. Wildgruber, and R. A. Wever. 1986. "Meal Timing in Humans During Isolation Without Time Cues." *Journal of Biological Rhythms* 1:151-162.

Broughton, R., and Q. Ghanem. 1976. "The Impact of Compound Narcolepsy on the Life of the Patient." In P. Passouant, ed. *Narcolepsy.* New York: Spectrum.

Carskadon, M. A., W. C. Dement, M. M. Mitler, T. Roth, P. R. Westbrook and S. Keenan. 1986. "Guidelines for the Multiple Sleep Latency Test (MSLT): A Standard Measure of Sleepiness." *Sleep* 9:519-524.

Green, J., C. P. Pollak and G. P. Smith. 1987. "The Effect of Desynchronization on Meal Patterns of Humans Living in Time Isolation." *Physiology and Behavior* 39:203-209.

Mitler, M. M., J. van den Hoed, M. A. Carskadon et al. 1979. "REM Sleep Episodes During the Multiple Sleep Latency Test in Narcoleptic Patients." *Electroencephalography in Clinical Neurophysiology* 46:479-481.

Pollak, C. P., M. L. Moline and D. R. Wagner. 1990. "Cognitive and Motor Performance in Narcoleptic Subjects Living in Temporal Isolation." Paper presented at Annual Meeting, Northeastern Sleep Society, March 31-April 1, 1990, Boston, MA.

Pollak, C. P. and J. Green. 1989. "Circadian Meal Timing in Narcoleptic Subjects Living in Time Isolation (Abst.)." Northeastern Sleep Society, March 31-April 1, White Plains, NY.

Pollak, C. P., D. R. Wagner and M. L. Moline. 1990. "Sleep Duration and Sleep Need in Narcoleptic Subjects Living Without Temporal Cues." Submitted to *Archives of Neurology.*

Rechtschaffen, A. and A. Kales. 1968. *A Manual of Standardized Terminology, Techniques and Scoring System for Sleep Stages of Human Subjects.* United States Public Health Service, U.S. Government Printing Office, Washington, DC.

Rosenthal, L. D., L. Merlotti, D. K. Young, F. J. Zorick, R. M. Wittig, T. A. Roehrs and T. Roth. In press. "Subjective and Polysomnographic Characteristics of Patients Diagnosed with Narcolepsy." *General Hospital Psychiatry.*

Wever, R. A. 1979. *The Circadian System of Man: Results of Experiments Under Temporal Isolation.* New York: Springer-Verlag NY, Inc.

A Counseling Service for Narcolepsy: A Sociomedical Model

Meeta Goswami

Narcolepsy is a sleep disorder of neurological origin with a strong genetic basis. Its principal features are excessive daytime sleepiness and cataplexy (muscular paralysis precipitated by strong emotion or stress). Auxiliary symptoms include sleep paralysis, hypnagogic hallucinations, automatic behavior, and disturbed nocturnal sleep. The condition is treated with central nervous system stimulants for daytime sleepiness and tricyclic antidepressants for cataplexy. The cure for this treatment is not presently known.

The multiple effects of narcolepsy on the life of affected individuals and their families are well documented. Deleterious impact on work, education, driving record, and interpersonal relationships are reported by Broughton et al. (1981) and Kales et al. (1982). The wide-ranging effects of this condition on marital life and employment and a perceived need on the part of patients for psychosocial support (Goswami, Glovinsky and Thorpy 1987) demonstrate the importance of developing a program to fulfill these needs.

This presentation attempts to elucidate an integrative model for patient management in narcolepsy. The model explicates the roles of the physician and the counselor and specifies the medical, genetic and general counselling components pertaining to narcolepsy.

Meeta Goswami, PhD, MPH, is Director, Narcolepsy Project, Sleep/Wake Disorders Center, Montefiore Hospital and Medical Center, Bronx, NY.

Initiated in 1985, and following several experiments, this sociomedical model is being implemented at the Narcolepsy Project, Montefiore Medical Center. The mission of the program is to provide comprehensive and integrated care to patients and to establish a synergistic link between the social, psychological, spiritual, and biomedical aspects of health. It is funded and supported by the New York State OMRDD.

The author is grateful to Joyce Howard and Mihir Goswami for editorial assistance.

This concept in program development may be applicable to other chronic illnesses as well.

Traditionally, the model for counseling has followed the medical model of disease causation and medical care delivery, where the physician is the primary and predominant source of care. In this traditional model, the doctor-patient relationship is asymmetrical and counseling is directive. Communication generally flows from physician to patient, and the physician's emphasis is on providing medical information and advice on the diagnosis, treatment, and genetic factors related to the patient's condition. Here, the patient is perceived as a passive receiver of services. How he perceives his illness, what impact it may have on his life, or what other support services, if any, may be needed, is often not known (Bloom and Wilson 1972).

The sociomedical model of counseling proposed here recognizes that a series of factors, which may be biomedical, social, and psychological, may contribute to, or result in, a presenting illness. Therefore, interpersonal and socioenvironmental factors are important considerations in the development and delivery of medical services. In this model, communication is nondirectional, and emphasis is placed on receiving feedback from patients as well as providing them with information and involving the patient in the decision-making process (Hsia et al. 1979).

The counseling process as defined here includes imparting information about the condition as well as providing support and/or therapy when social or psychological problems are manifested. Counseling entails:

- Defining the problem;
- Setting goals;
- Developing a set of alternative solutions;
- Prioritizing solutions;
- Developing a plan of actions within a specific time frame;
- Implementing actions;
- Assessing outcome.

Our experience in program development shows that counseling, generally speaking, and more specifically, the supportive dimension of counseling, requires time and excellent communication skills. With increasing technological advancement, a physician must keep in touch with the latest information in his area of expertise. Thus, he or she may lack the time and/or the skills and perhaps even the aptitude for comprehensive counseling. Therefore, an alternative model that would integrate the medical with the psychosocial aspect of care is needed.

This alternative model, described in this paper as a sociomedical model, is based on well-documented evidence that psychosocial factors influence (1) health status (Susser and Watson 1985; Freeman and Levine 1989; Kessler, House, and Turner 1987; Helsing and Szklo 1981; Johnson and Kaplan 1988), (2) utilization of health services (Verbrugge 1989; Mechanic and Aiken 1989; Leaf et al. 1985), and (3) compliance to a health regimen (Bartlett, Grayson and Barker 1984; Wilson and McNamara 1982; Davis 1968, 1971). This model requires a multidisciplinary approach to patient care management, encompassing medical, psychological, and socioenvironmental knowledge. To fulfill these requirements, a team approach to counseling is recommended. This proposal would call for a physician and a sociomedical counselor to provide the comprehensive array of medical, psychosocial and other support services that would be indicated for patient care. The team approach would provide greater cost efficiency than the traditional medical model, which required the physician to be both medical provider and counselor. The sociomedical counselor, with skills in communication and counseling as well as in public health medicine and evaluation techniques, would be an invaluable asset to the patient care management team. This professional, with a background in social science and public health medicine at the graduate level, followed by a year of training dealing with the specific illness (narcolepsy), would be an ideal counselor for such a service. A psychologist, sociologist, nurse, or social worker with special training in genetics, public health, and communication skills would be very effective in such a role. Ideally, this professional would be a generalist who is cognizant of and has training in the medical, social, psychological, and spiritual dimension of health. As described by many of our patients, the spiritual dimension of life plays an important role in the management of chronic illness, not only for the patient but for the family.

Professionals are socialized in long and intensive training periods to diagnose and treat patients in their areas of study. Consequently, they tend to restrict their observations in clinical practice to their areas of expertise, often remaining oblivious to whatever other issues and concerns the patient may present. Thus, a patient with multiple needs must seek help from several professionals. This tends to produce fragmentation of services, with no communication between providers or between providers and patients. Patients feel a sense of depersonalization and hopelessness in working with a complex system and eventually drop out from treatment. The end result is poor quality of care.

In the interest of providing high-quality care, the physician and sociomedical counselor must coordinate their activities and maintain open lines of communication so as not to duplicate services.

Tables I-IV outline the Narcolepsy Counseling Service components. The service is divided into five major components, each having a designated role for both physician and sociomedical counselor. The model incorporates specific needs in narcolepsy such as memory problems and time management. Implicit is the need to assist the patient by accessing and obtaining a wide array of services from professionals and agencies, and by helping him or her to develop effective interpersonal skills. On closer inspection of the model, it is clear that at each phase (component) of service, the medical aspect of the counseling is conducted by the physician. That psycho-socioenvironmental factors are manifested at each phase of the service demonstrates the need for a sociomedical approach to the counseling service.

A conceptual thread that runs through each phase of this model depicts the maintenance of continuity and comprehensiveness of care provided by one professional, a sociomedical counselor, who can provide basic information on social, psychological, nutritional, and genetic concerns. This level of information is generally satisfying to many patients with narcolepsy who do not desire to be treated as sick individuals but who do have one specific disorder and may be otherwise normal.

Patients with severe psychological or social problems requiring more intensive care may be referred to a specialist such as a psychologist, psychiatrist, or social worker. Referral for training and employment form important elements of this model. Continuity and comprehensiveness of care are provided by monitoring and assess-

A COUNSELING SERVICE IN NARCOLEPSY
(SOCIOMEDICAL MODEL)
ROLES OF PHYSICIAN AND SOCIOMEDICAL COUNSELOR

Table I.

DIAGNOSIS

Physician	Sociomedical Counselor
.Medical history	.Psycho-social history
.Physical examination	.Pedigree information
.MSLT, Polysomnographic tests	
.Interpretation of clinical findings	.Assessment of impact of diagnosis on patient and family (shock, denial, permanency, blame, guilt, self-image)

REFERRAL

.Screening/Laboratory Tests	.Preparation of patient
.HLA testing	.Clarification of expectations
.Other specialists	.Explanation of procedures

ing by outcome of care, and consistent follow-up. Behavioral indicators such as increased utilization rates are used to measure the need, as perceived by the patient, and demand for services. Important are factors such as:

1. The seriousness of the problem.
   What is the impact of the diagnosis on the patient and family?
   What is the impact of the problem on the life of the patient?
   What is the impact of the treatment on the quality of life of the patient?
   Do other concerns have higher priority than the presenting complaints in the life of the patient?
2. Who will prepare the patient and explain procedures for various follow-up tests?

3. What are the potential barriers to service utilization? Who will study these needs?
4. What support services are needed by the patient and/or family? Who will assess these needs?
5. What are the barriers to compliance with medical regimen? Who will promote compliance?
6. Who will be an advocate for the patient?
7. Who will provide spiritual counseling when needed?
8. Who is responsible for evaluation, follow-up, and coordination of services (including social and/or other outside support services)?

A COUNSELING SERVICE IN NARCOLEPSY
(SOCIOMEDICAL MODEL)
ROLES OF PHYSICIAN AND SOCIOMEDICAL COUNSELOR

Table II.

MANAGEMENT I
TREATMENT

Physician	Sociomedical Counselor
.Medical treatment	.Assessment of psycho-social issues related to medical management
.Follow-up	.Clarification of expectations Explanation of procedures
.Information/counseling on medical/genetic issues	.Interpretation/clarification of medical/genetic information
	.Assessment of barriers to patient compliance with medical regimen
	.Promotion of patient compliance
	.Provision of Services/ Referral for finances, home care, transportation, legal and other community services

A COUNSELING SERVICE IN NARCOLEPSY
(SOCIOMEDICAL MODEL)
ROLES OF PHYSICIAN AND SOCIOMEDICAL COUNSELOR

Table III.

MANAGEMENT II
Impact of condition/treatment
(adaptation)

Physician	Sociomedical Counselor
.Risk Prediction	.Risk Prediction

- not reproductive
- but accidents: Driving,
  home, work
	- not reproductive
	- but accidents: Driving,
	  home, work

.On-going counseling for medical aspects	.Counseling for effect of condition on education, social relations, marital life, work and psychological effects
.Management of adverse reactions of medications; recommend alternate modes of treatment	.Assistance in decision-making in regard to non-medical treatment and social aspects (nutrition, time-management, education, family life, work, memory)

	.Support - individual
	            family
	            group

	.Spiritual counseling
	.Referral...relevant community services, e.g. financial, recreation
	.Advocacy...education, work

These factors form the content areas for the sociomedical counseling model. As can be seen from the tables, the role of the physician and sociomedical counselor are complementary and supportive but very distinctive. Together they allow for a comprehensive approach to patient management and provide continuity of care. Also, they insure increased cost efficiency (of personnel time) and could result in increased utilization of services, greater patient compliance with treatment regimen, and improvement in the quality of life of the patient.

A COUNSELING SERVICE IN NARCOLEPSY
(SOCIOMEDICAL MODEL)
ROLES OF PHYSICIAN AND SOCIOMEDICAL COUNSELOR

Table IV.

EVALUATION
Treatment/Interventions

Physician		Sociomedical Counselor	
Follow-up:	Personal/Questionnaire/ Telephone	Follow-up:	Personal/ Questionnaire/ Telephone Psycho-social aspects
	Medical symptoms		.Patient compliance treatment regimen utilization of services

REFERENCES

Bartlett, E. E., M. Grayson, and R. Barker. 1984. "The Effects of Physician Communication Skills on Patient Satisfaction, Recall and Adherence." *Journal of Chronic Diseases* 37:755-764.

Bloom, S. W. and R. N. Wilson. 1972. "Patient Practitioner Relationships." In H. E. Freeman, S. Levine, and L. G. Reeder, eds. *Handbook of Medical Sociology*. Englewood Cliffs, NJ: Prentice-Hall.

Broughton, R., Q. Ghanem, Y. Hishikawa, Y. Sugita, S. Nevsimalova, and B. Roth. 1981. "Life Effects of Narcolepsy in 180 Patients from North America, Asia and Europe Compared to Matched Controls." *Canadian Journal of Neurological Sciences* 8:299-304.

Davis, M. S. 1971. "Variation in Patient Compliance with Doctor's Orders: Medical Practice and Doctor-Patient Interaction." *Psychiatry in Medicine* 2:31-54.

Davis, M. S. 1968. "Variation in Patient's Compliance with Doctor's Advice: An Empirical Analysis of Patterns of Communication." *American Journal of Public Health* 58(2):274-288.

Goswami, M., P. Glovinsky, M. J. Thorpy. 1987. "Needs Assessment and Socio-Demographic Characteristics in Narcolepsy." *Abstracts*, Fifth International Congress of Sleep Research, June 28-July 32. Copenhagen, Denmark, pp. 805.

Helsing, E. H. and M. Szklo. 1981. "Mortality After Bereavement." *American Journal of Epidemiology* 114(1): 41.

Hsia, Y. E. et al., eds. 1979. *Counseling in Genetics*. New York: Alan R. Liss, Inc. pp. 283-284.

Johnson, R. J. and H. B. Kaplan, 1988. "Gender, Aggression, and Mental Health Intervention During Early Adolescence." *Journal of Health and Social Behavior* 29:53-64.

Kales, A., C. R. Soldatos, E. O. Bixler, A. Caldwell et al. 1982. "Narcolepsy-Cataplexy." *Archives of Neurology* 39:169-171.

Kessler, R. C., J. S. House, and B. J. Turner. 1987. "Unemployment and Health in a Community Sample." *Journal of Health and Social Behavior* 28:51-59.

Leaf, P., G. L. Livingston, M. M. Tishler et al. 1985. "Contact with Health Professionals for the Treatment of Psychiatric and Emotional Problems." *Medical Care* 23:1322-1337.

Mechanic, D. and L. H. Aiken. 1989. "Access to Health Care and Use of Medical Care Services." In H. E. Freeman and S. Levine, eds. *Handbook of Medical Sociology*. Englewood Cliffs, NJ: Prentice-Hall, pp. 166-184.

Susser, M. W. and W. Watson. 1985. *Sociology in Medicine*. New York: Oxford University Press.

Verbrugge, L. M. 1989. "The Twain Meet: Empirical Explanations of Sex Differences in Health and Mortality." *Journal of Health and Social Behavior* 30:282-304.

Wilson, P. and J. R. McNamara 1982. "How Perceptions of a Simulated Physician-Patient Interaction Influence Intended Satisfaction and Compliance." *Social Science and Medicine* 16:1699-1704.

A Narcolepsy Patient Role Model

Joseph A. Piscopo

My name is Joe Piscopo. I am not related to the comedian of the same name. I am 45, married, with two sons ages 16 and 18. I am a native Californian, but I live in Oak Brook, Illinois, just west of Chicago. I have a bachelor's degree in computer sciences from the University of Illinois. I am a director and the current treasurer of the American Narcolepsy Association.

In 1969, at the age of 24, I founded a computer software company. It was called Pansophic Systems, Inc. Starting with only three employees and with $150,000 invested by my family and friends, Pansophic became a great success, with $115 million in sales, 1100 employees, customers in 60 countries and stock listed on the New York Stock Exchange! I retired from the company in 1987, at the age of 42, after 18 years as its Chief Executive Officer.

Of greater interest, perhaps, is the fact that I have personally contributed almost $2 million for narcolepsy research in the last three years. My desire is to stimulate new research efforts in diverse areas to find a cure or preventive treatment for narcolepsy. I also have narcolepsy. The purpose of this paper is to offer my own case history as a narcolepsy patient, hopefully to serve as a positive role model for other patients and others to emulate.

I have had narcolepsy since age 14, but I was not diagnosed until I was 20 and not treated effectively until I was 25. Unfortunately, that was after I had slept through most of my college classes. Between the ages of 16 and 25, I was the cause of 15 automobile accidents after falling asleep while driving. I was very fortunate to have graduated from college and really lucky to have survived some

Joseph A. Piscopo is Treasurer and Director, The American Narcolepsy Association, Oak Brook, IL.

165

very bad accidents without a scratch. Other narcopletics are not so fortunate.

In 1969, just after starting my company and just before I was married, I first visited the Mayo Clinic in search of narcolepsy treatment. I was directed to a neurologist on the clinic staff who had treated about 4000 narcolepsy patients in 35 years. He retired in 1982, but still maintains a private practice for narcolepsy patients in Rochester, Minnesota. I was diagnosed as having severe narcolepsy, with frequent sleep attacks, cataplexy, and most of the other classic symptoms of narcolepsy. The diagnosis was made after I gave a complete and detailed medical history, followed by a 10-minute pupillography test. That was all. To this day I have never taken a polysomnograph or a sleep study, nor have I had a multiple sleep latency test. I wonder often if these expensive and very inconvenient procedures are really necessary?

I propose a new standard for the effective diagnosis of narcolepsy:

> To be considered effective, diagnosis of narcolepsy should consist of the minimum number and extent of procedures necessary for the diagnosis of narcolepsy in the shortest time, at the lowest cost to the patient, and with the least disruption of the patient's lifestyle possible.

Even more important than effective diagnosis is the effective treatment of a narcoleptic patient. In 1969 at the Mayo Clinic, after my diagnosis for narcolepsy and a week of twice-daily visits with my doctor to monitor varying doses of methylphenidate (Ritalin) that I was taking without success, I was given a prescription for 100 mg. daily methamphetamine (Desoxyn), to be taken upon awakening. The results were remarkable! I was finally awake and alert.

I have continued the 100 mg. of Desoxyn daily, without increase over 20 years. I believe I am as alert as any normal person without narcolepsy. I am able to be productive and successful in life just like everyone else. There are negligible side effects from the high dosage of methamphetamine, including frequent dry mouth and indigestion from eating pizza! My blood pressure and pulse are checked frequently and are always normal. I take no drugs for my cataplexy. I have several cataplexy attacks daily, usually triggered by surprise or anger, but I have been able to limit the occurrences by controlling my personal style and social contacts. I haven't had an automobile accident since I was 25. I avoid driving late at night or long distances.

In my 18 years as chief executive officer of a high-tech growth company, I never required special treatment or accommodations due to my narcolepsy, although I generally avoided evening meetings or social affairs. At the time of my retirement, only my successor as C.E.O. was aware of my narcolepsy, as a result of my asking him for a contribution to narcolepsy research! I have no problem as a result of severe narcolepsy, although the drug laws have caused my doctor and pharmacist to be harassed periodically, and the cost of my medication has risen to ten times what it cost in 1969. I never take a daytime nap. In order for a narcoleptic patient to have a decent quality of life, special accommodations and naps on the job must be avoided. Our society is not able to provide special privileges in the work place. That is very unfortunate, but the way it is. I have never taken a "drug holiday," not even for a single day. What justification can be given for a patient to virtually withdraw from existence for two days out of seven? What benefit is gained from "drug holidays"?

I propose a new standard for the effective treatment of narcolepsy:

> To be considered effective, treatment of narcolepsy should consist of the minimum drug dose necessary to achieve and maintain a normal level of alertness throughout the day, without a need for special work place accommodations or privileges, and without a need for daytime naps or "drug holidays".

The Role of the Social Sciences in Medicine

Meeta Goswami

The role the social sciences has taken in the field of medicine in the past two decades has been impressive. Theory and methodology in the fields of anthropology, economics, political science, psychology, and sociology have been applied to the study of illness, the behavior of patients in regard to illness, the role of professionals in health care, and the study of organizations in which care is provided.

Medicine is a synthesis of several disciplines that applies clinical knowledge, skills and judgment in the care of the sick. Social science, on the other hand, deals with the disease process indirectly. Central to social science inquiry are interpersonal relationships and the perceptions and reactions of individuals to their psychological states and to their environment.

With changes in the delivery of the health care system, including technological advances, increase in the third party payment system and an increasingly sophisticated population, there is a stress on prevention, quality care and comprehensiveness of services. Furthermore, the evaluation of quality of care and quality of life, problems of manpower shortage and maldistribution of doctors, health care marketing and needs assessment are emerging areas of concern and interest in the health care delivery system. The study of these concerns and issues requires an increasing application of social science theory and methodology. Another notable change in the delivery of health care is the definition of illness, which has moved from a focus on disease to a focus on health, well-being, and happiness.

Meeta Goswami, PhD, MPH, is Director, Narcolepsy Project, Sleep/Wake Disorders Center, Montefiore Hospital and Medical Center, Bronx, NY.

There is a trend toward the concept of the "total patient." The patient is not to be looked upon as a diseased entity but as a total person as he relates to his social environment. Parsons (1951, p. 431) has defined illness as "a state of disturbance in the normal functioning of the total human individual, including both the state of the organism as a biological system and of his personal and social adjustments. It is thus partly biologically and partly socially defined."

In the context of this changing health care system and the definition of health, I would like to comment briefly here on the role in medicine of one particular social science, sociology.

Essentially, sociology concerns itself with the study of structural contexts in social institutions and the designation of statuses and roles. Some of these structures are the various systems of stratification, such as the ones based on social class, race, gender, age, ethnoreligious backgrounds, and marital status.

A major way in which sociology has contributed to medicine is the study of social factors as independent variables to explain morbidity and mortality. These social factors have included (in addition to those named above) social cohesion, social supports, and social stress in the study of various forms of morbidity, such as heart disease, suicide, alcoholism, and schizophrenia (Berkman and Syme 1979).

Gender is one social status on which a large body of research literature exists (Pearlin and Aneshensel 1986). The relationship between gender roles, morbidity and utilization of health services has generated considerable interest over the past decade. Overall rates of morbidity are similar in men and women, however, there is a difference between the sexes in rates of specific disorders (Robins et al. 1984). Women tend to have higher rates than men for disorders that involve subjective distress (Gore and Tudor 1973; Weissman and Klerman 1977). Whether these differences in rates reflect a higher rate of mental illness is questioned by some researchers (Gore 1978; Dohrenwend and Dohrenwend 1976).

Gender may determine the stressors to which people are exposed (Pearlin and Aneshensel 1986; Pearlin and Lieberman 1978). Furthermore, the effects of these stressors are likely to vary between the sexes, possibly due to differences in their roles (Pearlin 1975).

Men and women may differ in mobilizing their personal and mediating resources to deal with stress (Pearlin and Schooler 1978). Finally, gender may affect the ways in which stress outcomes are manifested; thus, women may show depressive symptoms, whereas men may show drinking and other behaviors (Aneshensel 1988).

The sociological concepts of roles, role-set and status-set (Linton 1936; Merton 1957) provide a useful set of tools to study work situations, family relationships, and the doctor-patient relationship. A role-set is an array of roles associated with each social status. Thus, the role of a doctor relates him to patients and co-workers. There may be potential conflict within the role-set, since the members of the role-set may have different social positions and different interests, values, and expectations. Parsons' classic analysis of the sick role several decades ago (1951) proposed an asymmetrical doctor-patient relationship in which the doctor transmitted information to a passive patient. Subsequently, Eliot Freidson (1970) and others pointed to the potential conflict in the doctor-patient relationship. This new perspective emphasized the dynamic nature of the interaction with both the doctor and patient trying to present their own definition and meaning of illness (Bloom and Wilson 1979).

A good doctor-patient relationship is not only mutually rewarding to both parties but, as some studies indicate, also affects the patient's compliance with treatment regimen and therefore treatment outcome. Thus, the doctor-patient relationship has important implications for quality of health care.

Providers of care must be sensitive to patients' perspective of illness, the impact of the condition on social functioning, and the effects of treatment (medications) on their lives. Medications may control the symptoms of a condition but may have adverse effects on the general health of individuals. Severe side reactions of certain medications may reduce levels of patients' compliance with medical regimens.

Finally, quality of life as a criterion to evaluate treatment interventions is a major development. This has occurred because of an increase in the prevalence rates of chronic illness, which parallels an increase in the aging population. Many of these conditions cannot be cured; however, the symptoms can be controlled with treatment. Also, attempts are being made to humanize health care and maintain the dignity of the sick individual. Quality of life as a concept draws our attention not only to the medical definition of health and illness but to a more complete social, psychological, and spiritual definition of the well-being of individuals—a broad social dimension that is the domain of sociology and other social sciences. In this context, social sciences have sought to develop health status indicators for the measurement of disability, dysfunction, and states of discomfort or dissatisfaction on the part of recipients of care.

The point to be made here is that structural contexts can affect the disease cycle. Although medical management of illness is necessary, it is by no means sufficient; the psychosocial management of illness by social science professionals, in conjunction with the care provided by physicians, should greatly improve the quality of care and the quality of life of our patients.

REFERENCES

Aneshensel, C. S. 1988. "Disjunctures between Public Health and Medical Models." Paper presented at the meetings of the American Public Health Association, Boston.

Berkman, L. F., and L. S. Syme. 1979. "Social Network, Host Resistance and Mortality: A Nine-Year Followup Study of Alameda County Residents." *American Journal of Epidemiology* 190:186-204.

Bloom, S. W., and R. N. Wilson. 1979. "Patient-Practitioner Relationships." In H. E. Freeman, S. Levine, and L. G. Reeder, eds. *Handbook of Medical Sociology*, 3rd ed. Englewood Cliffs: Prentice-Hall, pp. 275-296.

Dohrenwend, B. P., and B. S. Dohrenwend. 1976. "Sex Differences in Psychiatric Disorders." *American Journal of Sociology* 81: 1447-54.

Freidson, E. 1970. *Profession of Medicine: A Study of the Sociology of Applied Knowledge*. New York: Dodd Mead.

Gore, W. R., and J. Tudor. 1973. "Adult Sex Roles and Mental Illness." *American Journal of Sociology* 78: 812-35.

Gore, W. R. 1978. "Sex Differences in Mental Illness Among Adult Men and Women." *Social Science and Medicine* 12B: 187-98.

Linton, R. 1936. *The Study of Man*. New York: Appleton-Century.

Parsons, T. 1951. *The Social System*. New York: The Free Press.

Merton, R. 1957. *Social Theory and Social Structure*. Illinois: Free Press.

Pearlin, L. I. 1975. "Sex Roles and Depression." In N. Dalton and L. Ginsberg, eds. *Life-Span Developmental Psychology: Normative Life Crises*. New York: Academic Press, pp. 191-207.

Pearlin, I. I. and M. A. Lieberman. 1978. "Social Sources of Emotional Distress." In R. Simmons, ed. *Research in Community and Mental Health*. Vol. 1, Greenwich, CT: JAI, pp. 217-248.

Pearlin, L. I. and C. Schooler. 1978. "The Structure of Coping." *Journal of Health and Social Behavior* 19: 2-21.

Pearlin, L. I. and C. Aneshensel. 1986. "Coping and Social Supports: Their Functions and Applications. In L. H. Aiken and D. Mechanic, eds. *Applications of Social Science to Clinical Medicine and Health*. New Brunswick, NJ: Rutgers University Press, pp. 53-74.

Robins, L. N., J. E. Helzer, M. M. Weissman, H. Orraschel, E. Gruenberg, J. D. Burke, Jr., and D. A. Regier. 1984. "Lifetime Prevalence of Specific Psychiatric Disorder in Three Sites." *Archives of General Psychiatry* 41:939-58.

Weissman, M. M. and G. R. Klerman. 1977. "Sex Differences and the Epidemiology of Depression." *Archives of General Psychiatry* 34: 98-111.

SECTION IV:
POLITICAL AND LEGAL ISSUES
IN NARCOLEPSY

The Legal Aspects
of Narcolepsy

Clarence J. Sundram
Patricia W. Johnson

The purpose of this discourse on the legal aspects of narcolepsy is not to give you legal advice but rather to provide a *general* exposure to the laws dealing with disability. The legal rights and remedies available to an individual who suffers from narcolepsy and related sleep disorders are highly dependent upon the individual facts and circumstances of each case. The physician plays a key role in establishing the existence of the condition, the severity of the disabilities, and their impact upon the individual with narcolepsy. Armed with this information, an attorney can assess the legal rights and protections available to an individual afflicted with this disorder.

Clarence J. Sundram is Chairman, State of New York Commission on Quality of Care for the Mentally Disabled, Albany, NY. Patricia W. Johnson is Assistant Counsel, New York State Commission on Quality of Care for the Mentally Disabled.

This paper is intended to provide an introduction to the legal questions presented when a person has been diagnosed with narcolepsy and to discuss some of the legal considerations in determining the consequences of such a diagnosis. This paper is *not* intended to be an exhaustive treatise on all the legal aspects of narcolepsy. Legal questions may arise in a variety of contexts: fitness to stand trial on a criminal charge; narcolepsy as a grounds for divorce or its impact on obligation for child support and maintenance; eligibility for worker's compensation and unemployment insurance; professional malpractice and other tort claims.

This paper will address three areas of law which most commonly affect persons who have narcolepsy: first, the protections against discrimination in employment, based on this disability, that are available under state and federal laws; second, the major services and benefits that may be available from several programs created to assist people with disabilities; and third, the impact of laws governing driver's licenses and professional licensure upon an individual who has narcolepsy.

BACKGROUND

Narcolepsy[1] is defined as recurrent, uncontrollable, brief episodes of sleep, often associated with hypnagogic hallucinations, cataplexy, and sleep paralysis.[2] Hypnagogic hallucinations, which occur in 25-54 percent of narcoleptic persons, consist of a vivid dream-like state with false visual and auditory hallucinations.[3] Cataplexy is a sudden loss of muscle tone, usually precipitated by emotional stimulation such as laughter, anger, or fear. Approximately 60 percent of patients with narcolepsy experience episodes of cataplexy.[4] These episodes of cataplexy may last from a few seconds to as long as 30 minutes. Cataplexy is virtually pathognomonic or distinctively characteristic of narcolepsy, although its onset is often several years after symptoms of excessive sleepiness begin.[5] Sleep paralysis can occur with sleep onset or awakening. The brain wakes up while the body remains in rapid eye movement sleep. Thus, the individual appears peacefully asleep but can actually be experiencing a frightening dream.[6]

While narcolepsy's etiology is largely unknown, its classification as an impairment of the neurological system should not be disputed. This classification is important in consideration of whether particular laws concerning disability, such as the Rehabilitation Act or the Developmental Disabilities Act, apply to narcolepsy. Stedman's Medical Dictionary (1982), 24th Edition, defines neurology as the branch of medical science concerned with the nervous system and its disorder. The nervous system is the organ system which, along with the endocrine system, correlates the adjustments and reactions of an organism to internal and environmental conditions. It comprises the central and peripheral nervous system; the former is composed of the brain and spinal cord, and the latter includes all the other neural elements.[7] Common knowledge dictates that, if a person is unable to avoid the onset of sleep, the brain—that is, the neurological system—is suffering from an impairment.

The following references from the medical literature on the subject of narcolepsy support the conclusion that narcolepsy is an impairment of the neurological system, although the authorities differ in regards to whether the condition is also an impairment in the body's immune system.

Cataplexy and the other REM (rapid eye movement) sleep-related abnormalities, sleep paralysis, and hypnagogic hallucinations probably stem from a specific set of pathophysiologic conditions in the brain . . . Narcoleptics suffer from physiologic conditions that are associated with normal REM sleep but that are not noticeable to the healthy sleeper . . . Much of what we know about cataplexy comes from studies of cholinomimetic drug-induced cataplectic states in cats and canine narcolepsy, a naturally occurring neurologic condition in dogs that parallels human narcolepsy with respect to electrographic findings and response to drug therapy.[8]

Narcolepsy is a heritable neurologic disease linked to the HLA-DR2 phenotype.[9] (A phenotype is a property produced by the interaction of a body's gene with the environment.)

The high prevalence of the antigen (HLA-DR2) (an antigen is a substance inducing an immune response) in patients with narcolepsy provides a compelling argument for involvement of the immune system in the etiology of this condition.[10]

Taken together, the HLA phenotype data supports the notion of genetic predisposition to the clinical and polysomnographic signs of narcolepsy marked by the HLA-DR2 phenotype, but also suggest that narcolepsy may be acquired in patients who lack this phenotype. . . . The association of a class II antigen with a disease involving the central nervous system could be explained by unusual expression of DR antigens in a neurologic tissue. . . . Since narcolepsy is clearly a neurologic problem . . . these observations suggest that systemic autoimmunity is unlikely to underlie the etiopathogenesis of narcolepsy.[11]

Narcolepsy can be precisely diagnosed with modern polysomnographic (testing and behavioral observation) techniques, even though only 20 to 25 percent of individuals with narcolepsy suffer the complete range of symptoms.[12]

PROTECTION AGAINST DISCRIMINATION IN EMPLOYMENT

A number of different state and federal laws bar discrimination in employment on the basis of disability. The first question, in considering whether these laws offer any protection to a person who has narcolepsy, is whether narcolepsy is a "disability" or a "handicap" within the meaning of these laws.

From a medical perspective, the answer may be clear enough, but from a legal perspective one must examine the language of the particular statute, applicable regulations or policy guidelines adopted by agencies charged with administering the law, and interpretation of the statutory language both by administrative agencies and by the courts.

This paper will examine the protections afforded by the federal Rehabilitation Act of 1973,[13] and by the recently enacted Americans with Disabilities Act of 1990.[14] A number of states also have their own statutory prohibitions against discrimination. The New York Human Rights Law[15] is one such example that will be discussed.

The Rehabilitation Act of 1973

This statute was the first federal law barring discrimination on the basis of disability. It broadly defines an "individual with handicaps" to include a person who has:

(a) a physical or mental impairment that substantially limits one or more of the major life activities of such individual;
(b) a record of such impairment; or
(c) been regarded as having such an impairment.[16]

The first test of whether a person falls within this definition is establishing the presence of a "physical or mental impairment."

The federal regulations promulgated under Section 504 define physical impairment as "any physiological disorder or condition, cosmetic disfigurement or anatomical loss affecting one or more of the following body systems: *neurological*; musculo-skeletal; special sense organs; respiratory including speech organs; cardiovascular; reproductive; digestive; genito-urinary; hemic and lymphatic; skin; and endocrine"[17] (emphasis added).

As a neurological disorder, narcolepsy falls within this definition.

The second test of the definition of disability or handicap is to demonstrate that it "substantially limits" one or more major life activities.

Major life activities have been defined in regulations to include caring for oneself, performing manual tasks, walking, seeing, hearing, speaking, breathing, learning and working.[18]

The proof of substantial limitation may be offered by showing the difficulty persons with narcolepsy have in securing, retaining, or advancing in employment. This may be done by demonstrating an individual's job expectations and training, and the jobs from which he or she is disqualified. A detailed medical evaluation identifying the specific limitations and their effect upon the individual should be provided.

It is notable in this definition that a person may be treated as being handicapped for the purpose of protection from discrimination, *even though there is, in fact, no existing disability*, if it can be established that such a person either has a record of such impairment, or has a condition which others regard as an impairment.

In including paragraphs (b) and (c), it was the intent of Congress to attack the attitudes and prejudices that result in discriminatory treatment, regardless of whether the actual condition (e.g., facial scarring) is disabling.

The key nondiscrimination language of the Rehabilitation Act, Section 504, reads as follows:

> No otherwise qualified individual with handicaps . . . shall, solely by reason of his or her handicap, be excluded from the participation in, be denied the benefits of, or be subjected to discrimination under any program or activity receiving federal financial assistance. . . .[19]

To gain protection from discrimination under this law, the claimant must prove not only that he is an "individual with handicaps" but also that he is "otherwise qualified" for the position in question.

In *Southeastern Community College v. Davis*,[20] the Supreme Court made it clear that the words "otherwise qualified" mean that the person is able to meet all of the program's requirements *in spite of his handicap*. The burden is on the individual to show that he or she can perform the essential functions of the position with or without reasonable accommodations, without endangering the health or safety of others.

The next element of proof is that the denial of the position or promotion or the termination was *solely* by reason of handicap. In order to do this, it is important to show what the essential components of the job or position are and what potential accommodations could *reasonably* have been made to enable the individual to perform these essential components: for example, frequent breaks, flex time, job restructuring, and other changes that involve minor inconvenience and expense to the employer. The courts have made it clear that "reasonable accommodation," which the law requires, cannot be the elimination of an essential function or a substantial modification of the nature of the job, nor can it be an undue burden considering the overall size of the agency's program (*Southeastern Community College*).[21]

Finally, the individual must show that he or she was subject to discrimination; that is, that there is no good performance-based reason, other than the disability, for the decision.

If the plaintiff can make an arguable case of discrimination, then it is up to the employer to show that there were legitimate, nondiscriminatory reasons for the termination.

Perhaps the best way of understanding how these terms and concepts play out is to review a §504 case involving discrimination on the basis of narcolepsy.

In *Gard v. Chairman of the National Credit Union Administration*,[22] a case arising in Colorado, a plaintiff with narcolepsy brought a §504 complaint regarding his termination from probationary employment as a bank examiner. When interviewed for the job, the plaintiff told the employer that he had narcolepsy but that it was well-controlled by a structured physical routine and medication. He assured the interviewers that driving would be no problem, after being informed that driving was an essential part of the job. The plaintiff never requested any reasonable accommodation from the employer.

During his probationary period, he was terminated for unacceptable travel practices, inefficient time management, poor bank examinations, and an insubordinate attitude. (There was an altercation during a performance review interview.)

The court determined that the person was terminated not for narcolepsy but for deficient performance. In other words, it found that he was not "otherwise qualified," although clearly he suffered from a disability within the meaning of the law.

In another case, *Ross v. Beaumont Hospital*,[23] which arose in Michigan in 1988, a surgeon lost her privileges at the hospital named. She sued, alleging that her termination was due solely to narcolepsy, in violation of §504. Two medical experts testified that the plaintiff's narcolepsy was controlled by medication and that her surgical abilities had not been adversely affected by this disability. The court found, however, that the plaintiff was terminated for her abusive behavior, based on numerous incidents, and noted one incident where there was evidence of her falling asleep during a surgical procedure after medications had begun, although no patient had been injured due to her performance. Here again, the court found performance-based reasons for the plaintiff's termination, rather than discrimination on the basis of narcolepsy.

One of the factors that complicates determining whether the discharge is based "solely" on disability is that there is evidence that personality difficulties may be associated with narcolepsy.[24] Thus, some of the interpersonal difficulties that plaintiffs have encountered in the work place may in fact be a product of their disability. If so, and if the employee makes the employer aware of these disability-related problems, it may be incumbent upon the employer, in making "reasonable accommodations," to provide access to employee assistance programs, supervisory assistance and support to resolve such problems in the work place.

The Americans with Disabilities Act of 1990 (ADA)

Many of the key concepts incorporated in the ADA are drawn from the Rehabilitation Act of 1973, §504 of which banned discrimination against handicapped individuals "under any program or activity receiving federal financial assistance." But, under the Rehabilitation Act, handicapped individuals were not protected from discrimination by entities that did not receive federal financial assistance. The intent of the ADA, among other things, was to broaden this protection to most employers.

The definition of disability under the ADA is the same as "individual with handicaps" under the Rehabilitation Act. The Americans with Disabilities Act provides broad protections to individuals with disabilities, guaranteeing equal opportunities in employment, public accommodations, transportation, state and local government services, and telecommunication.

This law broadly bars discrimination against a qualified individual with a disability "because of the disability of such individual in regard to job application procedures, the hiring, advancement, or discharge of employees, employee compensation, job training, and other terms, conditions, and privileges of employment."[25]

A qualified individual with a disability "means an individual with a disability who, with or without reasonable accommodation, can perform the essential functions of the employment position that such individual holds or desires."[26] The law gives consideration to the employer's judgment as to what functions of a job are essential. If an employer has developed a written job description *before* recruiting or interviewing applicants, this description is considered evidence of the essential functions.

The ADA also requires employers to make "reasonable accommodations" and enumerates, among other such accommodations, job restructuring; part-time or modified work schedule; acquisition or modification of equipment or devices; appropriate adjustment or modifications of examinations, training materials or policies; and other similar accommodations.

Employers can be exempted from the reasonable accommodation requirement if they can demonstrate that such accommodations would impose "an undue hardship on the operation of the business."[27] "Undue hardship" means an action requiring significant difficulty or expense, considering such factors as the nature and cost of the accommodation; the financial resources and overall size of the business; the number of facilities and the structure and functions of the work force.[28] Effective July 26, 1992, this law covers all employers with 25 or more employees. Two years thereafter, coverage extends to employers with 15 or more employees.

Since the ADA is a new statute and no regulations interpreting it have yet been issued, the regulations and interpretations of the Rehabilitation Act of 1973 take on an added importance in understanding the scope of coverage of the ADA.

New York Human Rights Law

In addition to these two principal federal laws, a number of states have state human rights laws that protect against discrimination on the basis of disability. For example, the New York State Human Rights Law defines the term "disability" to mean:

> (a) a physical, mental or medical impairment resulting from an anatomical, physiological or neurological condition which prevents the exercise of a normal bodily function or is demonstrable by medically accepted clinical or laboratory diagnostic techniques; or

(b) has a record of such an impairment; or

(c) a condition regarded by others as such an impairment.[29]

As discussed earlier, narcolepsy would be covered as a physical or medical impairment resulting from a neurological condition.

This statute covers employers with four or more employees, public housing and accommodations, educational institutions, public services, amusements, and credit. Although it covers employers more broadly, in banning discrimination on the basis of disability, this law incorporates concepts similar to those contained in the Rehabilitation Act and the ADA:

> . . . in all provisions of this article dealing with employment, the term shall be limited to disabilities which do not prevent the complainant from performing in a reasonable manner the activities involved in the job or occupation sought or held.

The State Court of Appeals amplified this language in *Miller v. Ravitch*,[30] stating:

> The statute bars discrimination against an impaired individual who is *reasonably* able to do what the position requires. Unless it is shown that the employee's physical condition precludes him from performing to that extent, the disability is *irrelevant* to the job and can form no basis for denying him the position. (emphasis added)

The process of proving discrimination to gain the protection of this law would generally follow the path described earlier, although there is no explicit requirement for making "reasonable accommodations" in the state law.

SERVICES AND BENEFITS THAT MAY BE AVAILABLE

Several laws, both state and federal, provide programs, services, benefits, and entitlements for people with disabilities. Once again, to be eligible for these services and benefits, an individual who has narcolepsy must establish that he falls within the definition of disability in the particular statute. Generally speaking, these definitions are stricter and require demonstration of an actual, rather than perceived, disability, as their purpose is not to protect from discrimination but to create an eligibility for, or entitlement to, publicly funded programs. Among the programs and services that may be available to an eligible individual are short-term and long-term individualized service planning, treatment services, vocational rehabilitation, disability benefits, affirmative action and legal advocacy.

Developmental Disabilities Assistance and Bill of Rights Act[31]

This federal law creates eligibility for services through state developmental disabilities programs, and for legal and other advocacy services through federally-funded protection and advocacy agencies at the state level.

The law defines developmental disability to mean a severe, chronic disability of a person which:

    (a) is due to a mental and physical impairment or combination of both;
    (b) begins before the person reaches age 22;
    (c) is likely to continue indefinitely;
    (d) results in substantial limitations in three or more of the following major life activities:
        1. self care;
        2. speaking and understanding;
        3. learning;
        4. mobility;
        5. self-direction;
        6. capacity for independent living; and
        7. economic self-sufficiency;
    (e) reflects the person's need for a combination of special care, treatment and other services which are individually planned and coordinated.[32]

Many of the concepts in this definition are similar to those discussed earlier (e.g., physical impairment, substantial limitations), but there is a higher level of severity. The applicant must be able to demonstrate through medical and other evidence that the substantial limitations affect *three or more* of the enumerated major life activities; that the age of onset was prior to 22; and that the severe, chronic disability is likely to continue indefinitely.

This law, however, creates merely an eligibility for individually planned and coordinated special care, treatment and other services; it does *not* create an entitlement. Similarly, people who are "developmentally disabled" are eligible for legal and nonlegal advocacy services from independent protection and advocacy agencies which each state and territory is required to have.[33] These advocacy agencies may assist them in pursuing remedies for discrimination, seeking benefits and services for which they are eligible or to which they may be entitled.

State Mental Hygiene Law

In addition to the federal Developmental Disabilities Act, states have statutes governing eligibility for services from the state's developmental disabilities service system. As an example, New York's law also creates eligibility for services and defines a "developmental disability" as a disability of a person which:

(a) is attributable to mental retardation, cerebral palsy, epilepsy *neurological impairment* or autism;
(b) originates before such person attains age *22*;
(c) has continued or can be expected to continue *indefinitely*; and
(d) constitutes a *substantial handicap* to such person's ability to function normally in society.[34]

The Rehabilitation Act of 1973

Title I of this Act authorizes a federal/state program to provide comprehensive vocational rehabilitation services to individuals with disabilities. This part of the Act defines "individual with handicaps" to mean a person who "(a) has a physical or mental disability which for such individual constitutes or results in a substantial handicap to employment and (b) can reasonably be expected to benefit in terms of employability from vocational rehabilitation services."[35]

Such services include any goods or services necessary to render an individual with handicaps employable, including evaluation and diagnostic services, medical services, counseling, referral and placement, training and prosthetic devices or other technological aids.

The Act provides a list of disabilities potentially covered by the definition of "severe handicaps," including neurological disorders.

If eligible for services under this Act, a person also is eligible for assistance from a Client Assistance Program, which is intended to provide legal and other advocacy to assist in obtaining necessary services.

Two other provisions of the Rehabilitation Act require affirmative action to increase job opportunities for disabled persons. Section 501 requires federal departments and agencies to implement affirmative action plans to encourage the hiring, placement, and promotion of disabled individuals. §503 requires businesses receiving federal contracts of $2500 or more to take affirmative action to employ and advance qualified individuals with disabilities.

Social Security Programs

The Social Security Disability Income program (SSDI)[36] provides basic income support to disabled persons unable to work as a result of their impairment. A worker, who has paid into the social security system, is eligible for benefits if he can prove an inability to engage in "substantial gainful activity" because of a medically certified physical or mental condition which is expected to last for at least 12 months or result in death.[37]

The Supplemental Security Income program (SSI) uses the same standard of disability as SSDI and provides monthly financial support to aged, blind, and disabled persons who have limited income and resources.[38]

Individuals who are disabled and who cannot engage in substantial, gainful activity are eligible for benefits from SSI and SSDI. Generally speaking, narcolepsy is treated as the statutory equivalent of epilepsy, which is a listed impairment in Federal regulations and is therefore entitled to a presumption of impairment.[39] Thus, people with narcolepsy have been found eligible for benefits.[40]

For example, an electrician who suffered three sleep attacks a day was found eligible for Social Security Disability insurance benefits.[41] However, if the disability is controlled by medication, benefits may be denied.[42]

To establish both the disability and its severity, the physician's testimony and evidence of laboratory tests are usually necessary. Relying upon a client's testimony alone is usually not sufficient. More information on these benefits may be found in *"Guide for Persons Seeking Disability Benefits Because of Narcolepsy"* prepared by the American Narcolepsy Association.

LICENSING

In general, the requirement of a license implies not only an authorization but a command to licensing agencies to take reasonable steps to see that the applicant is a fit and proper person to engage in the licensed business or profession. The law typically gives broad discretion to licensing authorities to require proof of fitness and their decisions to grant or withhold a license will generally be respected unless it can be shown that the decision was arbitrary and capricious, or in plain violation of law.

Driver's Licenses

These general principles apply to the issuance of a driver's license. The Commissioner of Motor Vehicles may require proof of fitness for people who have experienced a loss of consciousness. This requirement specifically applies to people who are not aware of their surroundings or are unable to receive or react to sensory impressions as a result of narcolepsy. New York State's motor vehicle regulations[43] require for proof of fitness for driver's license, a physician's statement that:

(a) the individual has *not* experienced a loss of consciousness in the last year; or

(b) the individual *has* experienced a loss of consciousness within the past 12 months due to a change in medication; or

(c) the individual *has* experienced a loss of consciousness within the last 12 months but this condition will not interfere with safe operation of a vehicle; and the Commissioner, acting after a recommendation from *his* medical consultant, finds no reason to disagree.

These regulations rely heavily upon medical evidence of the nature and severity of the disability, as well as of the degree to which it is controllable and of the extent to which it will interfere with the safe operation of a vehicle. The Commissioner of Motor Vehicles must accept the medical opinions unless he finds reason to disagree.

Professional Licenses

Here again, licensing agencies have broad discretion to determine fitness to practice businesses and professions and to require proof of fitness.

The nondiscrimination provisions of §504 do not cover State professional licensing unless there is some Federal financial participation.

The broad language of the ADA, prohibiting discrimination by a "public entity," including state agencies, that involves excluding qualified individuals with disabilities from participation in, or "benefits of services, programs or activities," probably encompasses licensing decisions. As such, it draws on the same concepts of "reasonable accommodation" to enable a person with a disability to meet the essential eligibility requirements for licensure.

There is a strong, evolving public policy against discrimination solely on the basis of disability, and a denial of a license solely on this basis could be found to be "arbitrary and capricious" unless there is a clear and strong link to the person's fitness to engage in the licensed profession or business.

As with employment, if the person is able to perform the duties of the profession with or without reasonable accommodations, he or she will probably be found eligible for a license.

On the other hand, if the nature of the disability substantially interferes with the performance of professional duties, to the point of rendering the person incompetent, licensure will be denied. In fact, such a severe disability may well be grounds for revoking a license once given.

CONCLUSION

Being afflicted with narcolepsy may create severe difficulties in day-to-day functioning. These difficulties may impair an individual's ability to work, sometimes seriously enough to make it impossible to hold a job. Legal protections are available under state and federal laws to bar discrimination, and to require reasonable efforts by employers to accommodate an employee who suffers from this disability. If the individual's condition is so disabling as to preclude substantial gainful activity, disability benefits may be available. If the onset of the disability requires a change in careers or assistance in meeting the demands of employment, services may be available from state vocational rehabilitation agencies. Finally, if the individual with the disability needs assistance in determining eligibility for any of these services or the scope of the protections available under the law (or in sorting through a legal maze!), legal and nonlegal advocacy services may be available from state protection and advocacy agencies, and client assistance programs.

Two points must be emphasized.

First, clear medical evidence must be provided to substantiate the disability, its severity, and the type of effects it has upon the individual. The results of polysomnographic testing should generally be made available. The physician should be able to state what capabilities or limitations the patient has, the extent of the disability and the conditions under which the effects of the impairment may be minimized. This medical evidence is likely to play a pivotal role in determining the legal consequences, rights, and entitlements of the individual.

Second, a lawyer should be consulted early for best protection of legal rights. While this paper attempts to present a simplified discussion of a number of different laws to familiarize nonlawyers with their key provisions, there are numerous legal considerations that have *not* been discussed. These considerations include essential elements such as the varying statutes of limitations which may bar claims entirely, the different procedures to invoke protection or benefits, the nature of the remedies available under each of these laws, the availability of administrative versus judicial proceedings, the varying scope of coverage, assistance in investigating a complaint of discrimination, the availability of attorneys fees, etc. Each of these factors plays a role in selecting a legal strategy for the most effective protection of the rights and interests of the individual client. A competent attorney should be able to examine these considerations and advise a client on the best legal course of action.

NOTES

1. Narcolepsy is also called Gelineu's syndrome and paroxysmal sleep and derives from "narco" and the Greek word "lepsis" — a taking hold, a seizure.

2. Dorland's Illustrated Medical Dictionary, 27th Edition (1988).

3. Cohen, F. L. "Narcolepsy: A Review of a Common, Life-long Sleep Disorder," 13 *Journal of Advanced Nursing* (1988) 546, 548.

4. Scharf, Fletcher, and Jennings, "Current Pharmacologic Management of Narcolepsy," 38 *American Family Physician* (1988) 143.

5. Cohen, *supra* at note 2, p. 547.

6. *Scharf, Fletcher, and Jennings, supra*, at p. 144.

7. Dorland's Illustrated Medical Dictionary (1988) 27th Edition.

8. Mitler, Nelson, and Hajdukovic, "Narcolepsy Diagnosis, Treatment and Management," 10 *Psychiatric Clinics of North America*, 593, 594.

9. *Id.* at p. 604.

10. Scharf et al., *supra*, at p. 144.

11. Rubin, Hajdukovic, and Mitler, "HLA-DR2 Association with Excessive Somnolence in Narcolepsy Does Not Generalize to Sleep Apnea and Is Not Accompanied by Systemic Autoimmune Abnormalities," 49 *Clinical Immunology and Immunopathology*, 149, 156.

12. Mitler, Nelson, and Hajdukovic, *supra*, at p. 596, 604.

13. 29 U.S.C. §701 *et seq.*

14. Public Law 101-336, 1990, 42 U.S.C. §12101 *et set.*

15. N.Y. Exec. Law, §290 *et seq.*

16. 29 U.S.C. §706(7)(B).

17: 45 C.F.R. §84.3(j)(2)(i).

18. 45 C.F.R. §84.3(j)(2)(ii).

19. 29 U.S.C. §794.

20. 442 U.S. §397 (1979).

21. *Id.*

22. 1989 WL (Westlaw) 48037 (D. Col. May 1989).

23. 687 F. Supp. 1115 (E.D. Mich. 1988).

24. See, e.g., *Stout v. Heckler*, 579 F. Supp. 237 (D. Idaho, 1985).

25. 42 U.S.C. §12112(a).

26. 42 U.S.C. §12111(8).

27. 42 U.S.c. §12112(b)(5)(A).

28. 42 U.S.C. §12111(10).

29. N.Y. Exec. Law §292, subd. 21.

30. 60 N.Y. 2d 527, 470 N.Y.S. 2d 558, 45 N.E. 2d 1235 (N.Y., 1983).

31. Public law 94-103, as amended, 42 U.S.C. §6000, *et seq*.

32. 42 U.S.C. §6001(5).

33. 42 U.S.C. §6042.

34. NYS Mental Hygiene Law, Section 1.03, subd. 22.

35. 29 USC §706(8)(A).

36. Title 11 of the Social Security Act, 42 U.S.C. §401 *et seq*, 20 CFR Part 404.

37. 42 USC §416(i).

38. 42 USC §1382c(a)(3); 20 CFR Part 416.905.

39. *Winans v. Bowen*, 853 F. 2d 643 (9th Cir. 1987) as amended 1988.

40. *Stout v. Heckler*, 579 F. Supp. 237 (U.S.D.C. Idaho, 1984); (W.D. Ark., 1987); *Boeltz v. Bowen*, 648 F. Supp. 733 (W.D. Pa., 1986).

41. *Winans v. Bowen, supra*.

42. *Van Wormer v. Sec. of HHS*, 875 F. 2d 869 (6th Cir. 1989) (this decision is unpublished but is available on Westlaw. There are restrictions to its use in court); *Chesterfield v. Sec. HHS* 816 F. 2d. 678 (6th Cir., 1987).

43. 15 NYCRR Part 9.

Can Narcolepsy Be Eradicated in This Millennium?

William Dement
Emmanuel Mignot

The Congress of the United States has designated the 1990s, leading into the next millennium, as the Decade of the Brain. During these ten years, scientific efforts to understand the human brain are to be greatly enhanced. This is perhaps more audacious than any societally mandated research focus in the history of mankind. Society has indeed confronted such great problems as the ultimate structure of matter and energy and the molecular biology of inheritance and of genetic regulation of the organism, but understanding the brain and the mind is far beyond this, and we may wonder if humans even possess the capacity. We are beginning to accumulate knowledge about the development of a complex nervous system, and of the many ways in which nerve cells can and do interact. Beyond our conception at the present time are the workings of learning and memory, and beyond that, we don't have a glimmer about how the organic structural nervous system gave rise to human consciousness. Some thinkers have assumed that the unimaginably complex interplay of sensory input, sensation, and perception, and the elaboration of complex motor responses, carries the inevitable seed of, or emerging property of, consciousness.

It is within this context that we explore the mystery of the sleeping brain. We remain awed by our experiences in the dream world.

William Dement, MD, PhD, ACP, is Director, Sleep Disorders Center, Stanford University Medical School and Chairman, Board of Governors, Association of Professional Sleep Societies, Stanford, CA. Emmanuel Mignot is affiliated with the Sleep Disorders Center, Stanford University Medical School, Stanford, CA.

Many anthropologists think that primitive man's attempt to account for dreaming and the contradiction that it presents gave rise to the notion of a spiritual or noncorporeal world. In other words, the concept of a spirit or soul or life force was the only way to account for neurological events and the permanent departure of some life force at the time of death. The discovery of rapid eye movements in the 1950s and the description of a new state of sleep, which was associated with the most vivid experiences of the dream world, greatly increased scientific and psychological interest. However, as we approach the Decade of the Brain, we find only the barest mention of sleep research in the documents and plans of the leading institute — The National Institute of Neurological Diseases and Stroke (NINDS) — and none at all in the planning documents of the National Institute of Mental Health.

Fortunately for sleep research and narcolepsy research, the rise of sleep disorder medicine in the past two decades has provided a new platform from which to advocate that the Decade of the Brain also be the Decade of the Sleeping Brain. The advocacy of the sleep disorders community has persuaded the Congress of the United States to legislate another effort, the National Commission on Sleep Disorders Research. This Commission will also promote research on the sleeping brain, and everything that derives therefrom, and will emphasize the research opportunities and the excitement that effectively exploring the *terra incognito* of sleep will entail.

A major reason for taking note of the Decade of the Brain is that sleep is in the brain, and narcolepsy is a disorder of the neurons and neurochemicals in the human cerebrum that are responsible for the generation of NREM sleep and REM sleep, and for the regulation of the circadian and homeostatic timing and quantification of sleep and wakefulness. Of course, narcolepsy is not the only sleep disorder. However, it is a quintessential sleep disorder, and as such, is an illness whose understanding is likely to yield enormous additional benefits for humanity beyond the crucial benefit of actually eradicating the illness. The research effort to understand the activities and purposes of sleep is vastly underfunded and neglected. Given the role that sleep plays in our daily lives, and given the magnitude and scope we can now assign to all the sleep disorders as well as to narcolepsy, current research support is ridiculously small.

In terms of doing something about it, to paraphrase Dickens, "It is the best of times, it is the worst of times." The research opportunities, the visibility, and the political effectiveness of the sleep research community and the patient volunteer groups has never been higher. On the other hand, the availability of National Institutes of Health funding has never been lower. There are two pathways that patients with narcolepsy have followed as they have attempted to promote narcolepsy research. One is an alliance with other "rare" diseases, and the second is some attempt to work through the orphan drug program for the development of better treatments. My career has led me to advocate the third pathway, and this is a total alliance with sleep research and sleep disorders medicine. I firmly believe that understanding sleep mechanisms will aid in understanding narcolepsy and, even more passionately, that understanding narcolepsy will lead to a better understanding of sleep and its various functions.

Although we can pat ourselves on the back for the research and other opportunities that have been created, we must always adjust our perspective to the world view. It is a simple, bold truth that sleep and its disorders should be half of everything. In general, we are either awake or we are asleep. Against this simple, bold reality, the support of sleep research and narcolepsy research is pitiful. The immediate political challenge is to go from essentially nothing to a remedial and permanent something. Even in the worst of times, it should be possible to accomplish this if the effort is politically effective and scientifically sound.

The statement that most exemplifies the current state of affairs is one made by Joe Piscopo, a member of the American Narcolepsy Association, on June 7th, 1988 in testimony before the Health Appropriations Subcommittee: "Mr. Chairman, the few narcolepsy studies that are now being conducted within NINDS are very important, but clearly the greater federal focus must be placed on narcolepsy research. I have personally funded more narcolepsy research over the last three years than the National Institutes of Health — a total of almost $2 million. It is just not enough. A disorder that affects more than 200,000 people in such a way should be the object of a higher level of federal funding for research."

Although federal funding has not yet increased substantially, the visibility of sleep disorders has, and this is the crucial first step. As a consequence of such efforts, both the House and Senate have urged that a greater level of NINDS resources be dedicated to narcolepsy research, and that NINDS explore methods of establishing a better focus throughout NIH and the scientific community on these disorders, and to organize a symposium on narcolepsy research. In addition, "in conjunction with the Decade of the Brain commencing on January 1, 1990, the Assistant Secretary for Health is directed to work with the National Academy of Sciences/Institute of Medicine to sponsor a symposium to bring together leading scientists from all relevant disciplines to discuss the state of the art and discourse upon short- and long-term goals. Funding shall be provided from available funds, including the 1% evaluation set aside." Finally, the National Commission on Sleep Disorders research is almost in existence. The numerous rumors we have heard lead us to believe that at least four of the Commissioners will have a documented and even intense interest in narcolepsy research and the diagnosis and treatment of patients with narcolepsy.

While these things I have noted may lead to benefits and better treatments in the distant future, they are not specifically directed to a better life for the sleepy patient right now. This, it seems to me, must come from an emphasis on narcolepsy and sleepiness in the training of sleep disorders physicians, and in the training of medical students, and in an enhancement of public awareness. Here again, the political and public relations mileage will come from linking the problems of narcolepsy to the general problems of sleep loss and fatigue. The final issue that should be very clear is that we should support neuroscience research in general because the techniques of neuroimmunology, molecular neurobiology and neuroscience can be profitably applied and, indeed, are absolutely necessary to understand the sleeping brain. However, it is not the techniques of research that concern us. These are being developed and advanced in admirable manner. It is how they are applied and the goals of the research.

What follows is a brief summary of the current understanding of narcolepsy held by researchers around the world. A number of outstanding research opportunities have been created by the ongoing research currently in progress on the genetic aspects of this illness.